An Introductory Course
In The Care and Prevention
of Athletic Injuries

Basic
Athletic
TRAINING

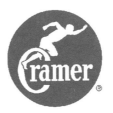

Cramer Products Inc.
P.O. Box 1001
Gardner, Kansas 66030

D1446133

ACKNOWLEDGEMENTS

Cramer Products would like thank the following professionals for providing invaluable assistance in writing, editing and reviewing the material contained in Basic Athletic Training, Second Edition:

Ms. Kimberly Babeu, Head Athletic Trainer
Marana High School, Tucson, AZ

Ms. Deidre Leaver Dunn, Research Assistant
The University of Alabama, Tuscaloosa, AL

Mr. David Bayes, Head Athletic Trainer
Boyd County High School, Ashland, KY

Mr. Ed Mizicko, Head Athletic Trainer
John Jay High School, San Antonio, TX

Ms. Patricia Billingslea, Head Athletic Trainer
Dunbar Senior High School, Washington, D.C.

Mr. Ben Velasquez, Doctoral Candidate
Middle Tennessee State University, Murfreesboro, TN

Mr. Rodney Brown, Manager, DCH Sports Medicine
Northport, AL

In addition, Cramer would like to acknowledge the efforts of Beverly Stevens, Mary Horvatin, Scott Holzrichter, Greg Unruh, A.T., C., and Tom Wealand, without whose efforts the production of this textbook would not have been possible.

ISBN 1-889366-01-3

Preface

Basic Athletic Training, Second Edition, is written and edited by Certified Athletic Trainers as a comprehensive introduction to current philosophies, procedures and practices relating to the prevention and care of athletic injuries. Designed to be used either as a classroom textbook or a self-study course, Basic Athletic Training, Second Edition, will prove to be challenging and rewarding for the beginning and intermediate athletic training students. It will also serve as an important refresher course and reference guide for coaches and other individuals concerned with the health and well-being of athletes.

The text is divided into 13 chapters and provides the reader with a step-by-step presentation of the training, responsibilities and techniques of the modern professional athletic trainer. For example, Chapter One, "Organization and Administration," explains the make-up of the sports medicine "team," the student athletic trainer's responsibilities on that team, the organization of a functional athletic training room and provides information about professional careers in athletic training. Succeeding chapters are devoted to explorations of various body structures and how to prevent, evaluate and treat injuries which might be associated with those structures.

Included for the first time is information relating to preventing the spread of blood-borne disease and how to live with Occupational Safety and Health Administration's new rules governing the handling of biohazardous materials. Glossary and Terminology sections will help the athletic training student become familiar with the specialized language of sports medicine.

At the end of the text, the athletic training student will have learned the basics of athletic injury prevention, evaluation, treatment and rehabilitation and will have a working knowledge of the athlete's body and how to prevent, recognize, evaluate, treat and rehabilitate athletic injuries. Having gained this knowledge, he or she will be better prepared to assist the professional athletic trainers involved with his or her school's athletes and better prepared for advanced instruction in sports medicine and athletic training.

Basic Athletic Training
Table of Contents

Table of Contents (continued)

Table of Contents (continued)

Table of Contents (continued)

Chapter 1
Organization and Administration

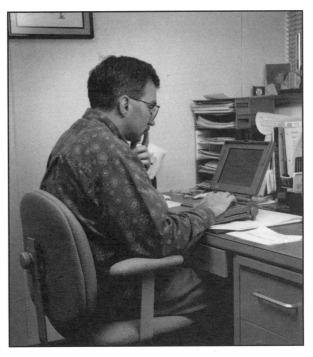

Educational Objectives

The learner should, at the completion of the chapter, be able to perform the following:

- Identify the components of the athletic training team.
- Understand the duties of the student athletic trainer.
- Establish the fundamental components of an athletic training facility.
- Recognize the National Athletic Trainers' Association (NATA) as the leader in this profession.
- Identify the educational programs for student athletic trainers.
- Understand the competencies of the athletic trainer.

What is athletic training? Simply stated, it is the prevention, recognition, evaluation, treatment, and rehabilitation of athletic injuries. However, implementation of the athletic training concept by a school system is not a simple action, for the program does not begin and end with the person designated as the athletic trainer. In fact, the program involves an entire team of people, including not only the athletic trainer, student athletic trainers and team physician, but also parents, coaches, the equipment manager, school administration and maintenance personnel.

Establishing an Athletic Training/Sports Medicine Program
Checklist for Safety in Sports

To establish an effective athletic training program school administrators should see that their school has the following:

- NATABOC Certified Athletic Trainers (ATC)
- Qualified coaches
- Qualified officials
- Required pre-participation physical examination
- Safe facilities
- Safe transportation to and from athletic events
- First aid kit
- Emergency medical plan
- Medical and dental insurance
- Injury notification system
- Accessible files such as injury reports and test results
- Adequate funding
- Adequate space
- Educational program

The Sports Medicine Team

The athletic training program starts with the individual appointed to supervise the care and prevention of athletic injuries—an athletic trainer. Before establishing an athletic training room and ordering supplies, the athletic trainer should perform a most important function: finding a team physician. The team physician will provide direct supervision of the athletic trainer.

Team Physician

With the team physician rests the success of the athletic training program. And, since athletic success is dependent on the health of the players, each team's success could be directly related to the

1

amount of time the physician can devote to the athletic training program. The team physician is captain of the medical team, which should include the athletic trainer, coaches, student athletic trainers, parents, and athletes. School administrators, the school nurse, and even game officials also share some of the athletic training responsibilities.

Duties and responsibilities of each member of the team are interrelated. Just as with any team, the medical team is only as strong as its weakest link. At the very least, a school should have a qualified team physician on the sidelines at football games or other contact sports. The team physician should be immediately available when emergency situations arise. Other team physician duties should include supervising pre-participation physicals and medical histories, clearing of players for return to activity after injury, working with the athletic trainer and student athletic trainers in further developing the athletic training program; and being on call for emergencies.

Other Medical Personnel
- Physical Therapists/Sports Therapists
- Massage Therapists
- Dentist/Oral Surgeon
- Emergency Medical Technician
- Cardiologist
- Gynecologist
- Internist
- Neurosurgeon
- Nurse
- Ophthalmologist/Optometrist
- Orthopedist
- Podiatrist

Other Personnel important to the Sports Medicine Team
- Equipment Manager
- Exercise Physiologist
- Nutritionist
- Strength Coach
- Sports Psychologist

Athletes
The athlete has the responsibility for keeping in good physical condition, practicing the techniques taught by the coaches, playing by the rules, and following the instructions of the coaches and athletic trainer.

Parents
The parents can assist in keeping their son or daughter healthy if they are kept aware of injury/illness by the athletic trainer or coach. The parents should be provided with information on nutrition and with recommended home treatments for injuries. When an athlete is injured, the athletic trainer must make the parents aware of the extent of the injury immediately.

Officials
Game officials must enforce the rules, monitor playing conditions, and cooperate with the athletic trainer and physicians when injuries occur and environmental hazards exist.

Coaches
Coaches have numerous athletic training-related responsibilities. They must plan practices that include conditioning and training of the athlete, and teaching of techniques and rules of their sport. These practices must be of reasonable duration, taking skill level, fatigue, and environmental conditions into consideration. Coaches are often responsible for selecting, fitting, and maintaining protective equipment. Additionally, supervision of practice and game facilities must be reviewed by the coaching staff. Coaches must update their education by attending clinics that review rule changes, skill development, first aid/C.P.R. and selected topics in athletic health care. Most importantly, the coach must place the athlete's welfare foremost. The coach must work closely with the team physician and athletic trainer in determining what is best for the athlete.

Note: If the school does not have an athletic trainer, these additional duties and responsibilities would then be assumed by the coach. See the "Athletic Trainer" section for a review of those duties and responsibilities.

Athletic Trainer

This person is vital to every athletic program. Without an NATA Certified Athletic Trainer (ATC), the responsibilities for the care and prevention of athletic injuries must be assumed by the coaching staff. Research studies have shown that injury rates will increase without an athletic trainer on site at practices and games. The athletic trainer serves as the liaison between team physician, coach, parent, and athlete. Communications regarding the health of the players must be channeled through the athletic trainer in order to have an efficient program. The athletic trainer, especially at the high school level, should maintain contact with parents regarding their son's or daughter's injury status and ability to return to active competition. Additionally, it may be necessary to notify the appropriate school officials (school nurse, physical education instructor, or principal) of limitations caused by an injury.

During the non-competitive seasons, the athletic trainer should work with the coaches on programs to improve the conditioning level of the team; devising specific conditioning programs for certain athletes, assisting athletes recovering from injuries, and monitoring athletes who need to increase their lean body weight or decrease their body fat. Additionally, the athletic trainer will assist the coaching staff and the equipment manager on the purchasing and reconditioning of protective equipment.

Under the team physician's direction, the athletic trainer will evaluate and provide first aid care, give basic treatments (ice/heat), outline rehabilitation programs, and apply protective/supportive techniques that will allow the athlete to regain an active lifestyle. Additional duties could include inventory/purchasing of supplies, completing medical/accident record forms, and treatments, etc.

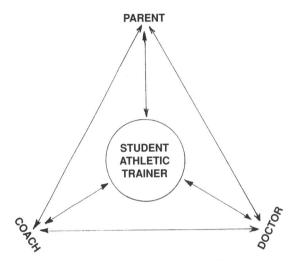

Members of the athletic training team are interdependent, with the student athletic trainer serving as an important liaison among coaches, athletic trainers, doctors, parents and athletes.

Student Athletic Trainers - Roles and Responsibilities

The duties of the final member of the medical team, the student athletic trainer, are the most difficult to define. For not only are student athletic trainers limited, in that they can be given little or no real responsibility, they are also constrained by the amount of time and instruction the coach, athletic trainer and physician can give them. If a student athletic trainer shows interest and ability in the job, the athletic trainer should do all he or she can to help the student develop.

Every student athletic trainer starts the same way: by maintaining a clean athletic training room/facility. Because various wounds are treated in the athletic training room, proper hygiene in this facility is critical. One reason is because of the possibility of cross contamination between bodily fluids and the various surfaces in the facility. Another duty assigned to a student athletic trainer would be inventory control, keeping track of supplies and equipment and informing the head athletic trainer when inventories are low. The student athletic trainer should have a checklist of supplies to have on the field or court for games, practices, or road trips. Packing of kits and other preparation activities are good duties for the student athletic trainer.

Additional duties might include preparing an electrolyte drink and taking it or water to the field; making sure there is enough ice, both for treatments and for water coolers; and making sure each athlete has weighed in before and after every practice and documented these weights on the weight charts.

Besides the weight charts, the certified athletic trainer or coach might give other record-keeping duties to a capable student athletic trainer. For example, daily treatments to athletes need to be recorded in a daily log and also in the athlete's medical file. As a student athletic trainer shows more initiative and competence, he or she may even become involved in taping, wrapping, changing dressings, giving minor treatments, and even some first aid. Besides the practical experience gained from working under the supervision of a certified athletic trainer or athletic coach, the student athletic trainer can also benefit from attending workshops and reading pertinent texts and publications.

Athletic Training Facility and Management

Establishing an athletic training room is very important. Athletic training room facilities at high schools vary from almost non-existent to those as modern and spacious as professional/college athletic training rooms. While everyone prefers good working conditions, facilities at some schools will always be less than ideal because of space or budget limitations. However, an athletic trainer will find a way to develop a program regardless of the limited facilities. Typical athletic training rooms include the following areas: electrical therapy, hydrotherapy (heat and cold application), taping, rehabilitation, administrative office, physician's examination area, and storage room. Listed on the following page is an outline of management items related to an athletic training facility.

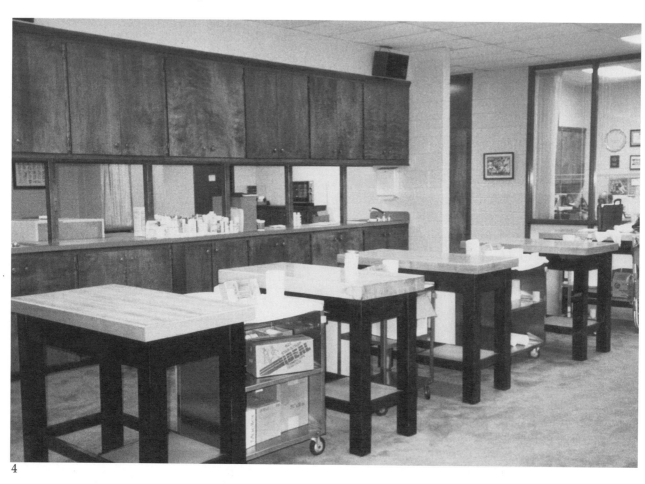

Athletic Training Facility Management

Office
- Vacuum the carpet
- Straighten shelves
- File any material in appropriate places

Taping Tables
- Stock all taping areas with supplies
- Wipe off top, front, and sides of taping tables with appropriate cleanser

Counter Area
- Clean top of counter
- Fill empty containers
- Restock shelves as necessary
- Straighten shelves
- Refill surgical trays with disinfectant solutions
- Clean surgical trays weekly

Treatment Area
- Clean off tops and sides of treatment tables
- Clean off tops of treatment machines and covers
- Check to see that the hydrocollator has sufficient water
- Check the paraffin bath
- Make sure sufficient towels are around the whirlpool area

- Disinfect and fill the whirlpools (HOT—100 degrees; COLD—55 degrees)
- Drain and clean whirlpools
- Fill ice cups and rotate those in the freezer
- Fill ice immersion buckets
- Make ice bags in the morning and before treatment
- Empty ice bags at end of day

Wet Area
- Clean sink, mirror, and stool
- Clean all coolers and place upside down
- Check supply of paper towels
- Clean whirlpools

Trash
- Empty into trash cans
- Put in new liners

Wipe Off
- Tables
- Hydrocollator
- Therapeutic modalities
- Rehabilitation equipment
- Ice machine
- Freezer
- Whirlpools

Supplies and Equipment - Athletic Training Facility

- Elastic wraps (2", 4", 6") and double length wraps
- Adhesive tape
- Alcohol, rubbing
- Hydrogen peroxide
- Band-aids
- Crutches
- Cups
- Disinfectant spray
- Elastic tape
- Eye wash
- Gauze pads (3x3, 3x4) sterile and non-sterile
- Antiseptic spray
- Ice machine
- Ice bags
- Pen light
- Refrigerator
- Rubber gloves
- Scale

- Scissors
- Soap
- Spine board
- Splints
- C-collar
- Tables (treatment, taping, examining)
- Tape cutters
- Thermometer
- Towels
- Water coolers
- Waste containers
- Whirlpool
- Blankets
- Face mask cutters (Trainer's Angel)
- Clock
- Hydrocollator (covers)
- Athletic training kits
- Broom and dustpan/trash can

In addition to the these items, the athletic training room must have those items that are mandated by the Occupational Safety and Health Administration (OSHA). These basically deal with bodily fluids and bloodborne pathogens.

Athletic Training Facility Management

Rehabilitation Room
- Wipe off all equipment, seats, and tables
- Make sure all equipment is in its proper place
- Sweep floor
- Make sure all modalities are turned off
- Make sure modalities are working properly (i.e., stim pads have adhesive backing)
- Check paper supply in isokinetic machine (if available)

Taping Area
- Restock tape remover
- Put new tape cutter blades in as needed
- Fill all containers
- Prepare heel and lace pads
- Clean up and sweep

Towels And Wraps
- Fold and put away clean towels and wraps
- Take dirty towels and wraps to laundry

Storage Room
- Straighten shelves
- Review inventory list
- Notify staff athletic trainers of limited supplies

Athletic Training Room
- Vacuum/sweep the floor

Records
- Review accident, injury and treatment forms
- File all medical records

Supplies for athletic training kits:

- Adhesive tape (1" to 1 1/2" rolls)
- Analgesics
- Antimicrobial hand wipes or soap
- Antacids
- Antibacterial/antiseptic cream
- Band-aids: regular, large, knuckle, fingertip, etc.
- Bandage scissors and/or tape cutters
- Biohazard bags
- Butterfly bandages or Steri-strips
- Contact lens kit
- Cotton tip applicators, Q-tips
- Elastic wraps (Ace wrap or tensor bandage): 3" and 6"
- Emergency information (athlete's home phone number, medical release forms, money, etc.)
- Eyewash, sterile solution
- Foot powder
- Heel cups
- Hydrogen peroxide
- Ibuprofen
- Instant cold pack
- Latex gloves
- Mirror with plastic holder
- Moleskin
- Mouth shield or protector
- Paper bag
- Pencil and paper
- Plastic bags for ice
- Povidine swab sticks or wipes
- Roller gauze

- Sterile gauze pads (3x3 inch)
- Saline solution/eye wash
- Scissors (bandage, heavy duty)
- Skin lubricant or petroleum jelly
- Sun lotion
- Tape adherent
- Thermometer
- Tongue depressors
- Triangular bandage or sling
- Underwrap

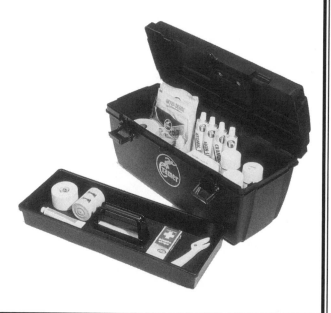

Athletic Training Room Rules

Once an athletic training room has been established, drafting of rules is very important. First, outline services that will be offered, specific times you will be open, and conduct allowed in facility must be reviewed. Remember, this is a medical facility and it should not be used as a gathering place. To prevent misuse, athletic training room rules should be posted and enforced. Among the common rules are:

- Co-educational facility
- Treatment provided only to student athletes
- Athletes should shower after activity before receiving routine treatments
- Equipment should be left in the locker room
- Loud music is not permitted
- Supplies and equipment will not be removed, except with permission of the athletic trainer

Rules can be adapted or added, depending on each school's situation.

Recordkeeping

In order to assure proper treatment of the athlete, careful records should be kept on all athletes. One form that every athlete should have in his or her file is a notation of his or her physical examination. The team physician may want to keep the original form at his/her office or in the school nurse's office. However, the athletic trainer should have a copy of the physical examination form or notations that are significant for the proper care of each athlete. The physical examination form should include not only the present condition of the athlete but past medical history as well.

Another form that is important in caring for athletic injuries is an accident-injury report form. This form should include the athlete's name, sport, date of injury, place of injury, time of injury, mechanism of injury, referral to physician, evaluation of injury, first aid given, and treatment and rehabilitation recommendations. An accident-injury report form is very important, particularly when the injury involves athletic insurance coverage and reporting. Insurance companies require accurate information

regarding the reporting of injuries. Check the insurance requirements at your school when designing your school's injury form.

The daily treatment form is another important document to be kept when treating injuries. There should be a place on this form for the athlete's name, the date, and what treatment or taping

INJURY REPORT

Dear Parent,
Your son/daughter, _____ (Name), has injured his/her _____ (Body Part), while participating in _____ (Event or Practice). As a result of the initial evaluation, it appears that he/she has _____ (Injury).
I have applied _____ (Immediate First Aid) and recommend that he/she _____ tonight. At this time I feel it is/is not necessary to see a physician. (circle)

I would appreciate it if you could help make sure proper treatments be administered, as this will help speed the healing and recovery process. It is also very important that I see _____ tomorrow, so that I may re-evaluate the injury. If you have any further questions, please feel free to contact me at the high school or at my home.

Sincerely yours,

Doug Nevitt
Athletic Trainer

PHHS — 778-2161
Home — 642-6357

EMERGENCY MEDICAL AUTHORIZATION

School District _____
Grade _____
Student Name _____
Address _____
Telephone _____
School Attended _____

Purpose — To enable parents and guardians to authorize the provision of emergency treatment for children who become ill or injured while under school authority, when parents or guardians cannot be reached.

PART I OR II MUST BE COMPLETED
PART I TO GRANT CONSENT

In the event reasonable attempts to contact me at _____ (phone number) or _____ (other parent or guardian) at (phone number) have been unsuccessful, I hereby give my consent for: (1) the administration of any treatment deemed necessary by Dr. _____ (preferred physician) or Dr. _____ (preferred dentist), or, in the event the designated preferred practitioner is not available, by another licensed physician or dentist; and (2) the transfer of the child to _____ (preferred hospital) or any hospital reasonably accessible.

This authorization does not cover major surgery unless the medical opinions of two other licensed physicians or dentists, concurring in the necessity for such surgery, are obtained prior to the performance of such surgery.
Facts concerning the child's medical history including allergies, medications being taken, and any physical impairments to which a physician should be alerted: _____

Date _____   Signature of Parent or Guardian _____
Address _____

DO NOT COMPLETE PART II IF YOU COMPLETED PART I
PART II REFUSAL TO CONSENT

I do not give my consent for emergency medical treatment of my child. In the event of illness or injury requiring emergency treatment, I wish the school authorities to take no action or to: _____

Date _____   Signature of Parent or Guardian _____
Address _____

procedure was received on that particular date. This form should be reviewed often when assessing the progress or lack of progress of an injury. It can tell you which treatment or taping procedure was successful in dealing with that particular injury.

The Fundamentals of Athletic Training

The "Athlete's Bill of Rights" states that every athlete is entitled to adequate conditioning and other injury prevention measures, proper treatment of injuries, and complete rehabilitation. The physician and athletic trainer could guarantee these rights. Programs for conditioning, injury prevention, and rehabilitation are best designed and supervised by a person with training in first aid, anatomy, physiology, and kinesiology; at the high school level, that person is usually a coach.

Having a team physician who is well qualified in sports medicine is important. Their assistance in reducing the risk of injury is vital. In the absence of a physician, the responsibility to give first aid treatment falls on the athletic trainer or coach. The student athletic trainer should be well qualified and provide assistance when needed. Individuals interested in becoming an athletic trainer should possess these characteristics: professional skills, knowledge required of athletic training, enjoyment of athletics, interested in each athlete's well-being, good fitness and personal health, common sense, and a willingness to complete assigned task. Avenues of employment for athletic trainers include employment in educational institutions (secondary and higher education), professional sports associations, sports medicine clinics, and hospitals.

National Athletic Trainers' Association
The Athletic Training Profession

In 1990, the American Medical Association recognized athletic training as an allied health profession. This endorsement is providing monumental benefits for the advancement of athletic training as a profession and for the professional development of the student athletic trainer. The National Athletic Trainers' Association (NATA) is the primary professional association of athletic trainers in the United States. Since the early 1960s, the NATA has assumed the leadership in establishing high standards for the education and certification of athletic trainers.

For more information on professional preparation or careers in athletic training you should contact:

National Athletic Trainers' Association
2952 Stemmons Freeway
Dallas, Texas 75247
1-800-TRY-NATA

Now that we know a little of what the profession of athletic training is and what it involves, we need to know who the people are that represent this exciting profession. The athletic trainer is a professional who is well educated to carry out on the tasks mentioned in the previous sections. A thorough knowledge of anatomy, physiology, physiology of exercise, psychology, first aid, cardiopulmonary resuscitation, nutrition, remedial exercise, and courses in athletic training are required in order to carry out these duties.

The National Athletic Trainers Association (NATA) is the administrative organization that dedicates its endeavors to the advancement, encouragement, and improvement of the athletic training profession. An athletic trainer who follows the educational procedures set forth by the NATA is then eligible to take an examination which, if successfully passed, entitles the athletic trainer to be a "Certified Athletic Trainer" (ATC).

Educational Programs: Curriculum and Internship

Student athletic trainers have the option to pursue one of two educational routes toward National Athletic Trainers' Association Board of Certification (NATABOC) certification. NATA approved Educational Programs provide a study in athletic training education which is approved by the Board of Directors of the NATA. Successful completion of an NATA-Approved Athletic Training Education Program requires no less than two years and includes 800 hours of athletic training experience under the supervision of a NATABOC Certified Athletic Trainer from the college or university sponsoring the NATA-Approved Program. Internship programs are designed to provide a practical education/work experience concept approach to gaining the knowledge and skills needed to fulfill the requirements for internship candidacy. Internship programs require the completion of 1500 hours of athletic training experience under the supervision of a NATABOC Certified Athletic Trainer.

Student athletic trainers, regardless of whether they complete a curriculum or internship program, must take one formal course in the following areas: anatomy and physiology, exercise physiology, kinesiology/biomechanics, personal health, basic athletic training, and advanced athletic training. To become a certified athletic trainer, individuals must:

- Complete either an internship or curriculum program
- Show proof of graduation from an accredited college or university
- Show proof of current certification in First Aid and CPR
- Show proof that at least 25% of their athletic training experience hours were attained in actual practice or game coverage with one or more of the following sports: football, soccer, hockey, wrestling, basketball, gymnastics, lacrosse, volleyball and rugby
- Obtain the endorsement of a NATA Certified Athletic Trainer
- Successfully pass the Certification Examination administered by the National Athletic Trainers' Association Board of Certification

NATA Competencies

The competencies enumerated in the document, "Competencies in Athletic Training", written and distributed by the National Athletic Trainers' Association Professional Education Committee (NATAPEC), have been identified as those necessary for effective functioning as an entry-level Certified Athletic Trainer (ATC). Results of role delineation studies conducted by the National Athletic Trainers' Association Board of Certification (NATABOC) in 1982 and 1990 served as the primary source for development of these competencies by the National Athletic Trainers' Association, Inc. Copies of the most recent Role Delineation Study may be obtained by contacting the NATABOC.

The Competencies in Athletic Training serve as a guide to development of educational programs and learning experiences leading to NATA certification as an athletic trainer and is intended to assist administrators, instructional personnel, and students in identifying knowledge and skills to be mastered.

The competencies included in the document are categorized according to the five major "domains" which comprise the role of the Certified Athletic Trainer:

- *Prevention of Athletic Injuries*
- *Recognition, Evaluation, and Immediate Care of Athletic Injuries*
- *Rehabilitation and Reconditioning of Athletic Injuries*
- *Health Care Administration*
- *Professional Development and Responsibility*

Although not stated as such, the competencies identified within each major domain are categorized according to the following commonly accepted method of classifying behavioral objectives:

- *Cognitive Domain (knowledge and intellectual skills)*
- *Psychomotor Domain (manipulative and motor skills)*
- *Affective Domain (attitudes and values)*

Conversion of the competencies into appropriately stated behavioral objectives and development of criteria for acceptable student performance is left to the discretion of instructional personnel.

Chapter 1 - Review Questions

Completion:

1. The student athletic trainer duties are limited, however, two important duties are _____ and _____.

2. Just as a coach, the student athletic trainer should maintain _____ certification.

3. The _____ _____ is the most important member of the athletic training team.

4. Every student athletic trainer starts by _____ the athletic training room.

5. Student athletic trainers can benefit by spending _____ and reading pertinent texts and _____.

6. A _____ _____ form should be kept to record all treatments given or tapings applied by the athletic training staff.

7. No matter what the athletic training room consists of, the athletic trainer must establish and enforce _____.

8. The most qualified individual to treat athletic injuries is a _____.

9. The majority of athletic trainers are employed at _____ _____.

10. The _____ is the primary professional association of athletic trainers in the United States.

11. A _____ is someone who has successfully passed the examination set forth by the NATABOC.

12. Internship programs require the completion of _____ hours of athletic training experience.

Short Answer:

1. List three important aspects of establishing an athletic training room:
-
-
-

2. Coaches play a very important part in the sports medicine program. List two things a coach should definitely know.
-
-

3. Name 5 of the 7 areas of an athletic training room.
-
-
-
-
-

4. List five employment situations where you could work as an athletic trainer.
-
-
-
-
-

5. List at least five medical personnel who should be included in the sports medicine team.
-
-
-
-
-

6. List 4 of the 6 requirements for becoming a Certified Athletic Trainer.
-
-
-
-

8. Items recommended by O.S.H.A. are used for what?

9. What is the "Athlete's Bill of Rights"?

10. What is the duty of the NATA?

11. What academic subjects are required in athletic training educational programs?

12. What role do parents play as a member of the sports medicine team?

13. Briefly explain the difference between the internship and curriculum programs in athletic training.

NOTES

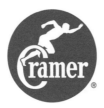

Chapter 2
Recognition, Evaluation, and Management

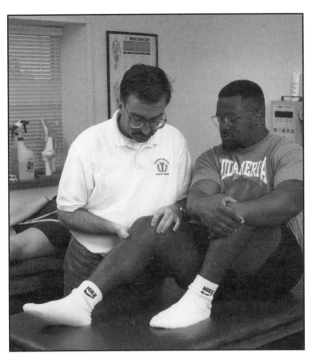

Educational Objectives

The learner should, at the completion of the chapter, be able to perform the following:
- Recognize the components of the injury evaluation format.
- Understand the fundamental treatment principles for athletic injuries.
- Identify the protocol in first aid and emergency care.
- Understand the steps in emergency transportation.

Recognition and Evaluation of Injuries

One of the primary functions of an athletic trainer is to determine (recognize) when an injury has occurred and how to evaluate the severity of that injury. The recognition of injuries is a process where the athletic trainer, either through direct observation or second hand accounts, determines the mechanism of injury and the probable causes for that injury. The recognition of the injury is the first step in the injury process. This is continued with the complete evaluation of the injury in order to determine the specific injury and the follow up management and treatment.

Evaluation Format: H.O.P.S.

First, calm and reassure the athlete; then begin your assessment with history, observation, palpation, and stress.

HISTORY
OBSERVATION
PALPATION
STRESS

Obtain a brief **HISTORY** regarding the mechanism of injury, location of pain, and sensations felt. Additionally, ask the athlete about prior injuries or surgical procedures at the current injury site. Ask questions about recovery from prior injuries.
- Mechanism of injury (how did it happen)
- Location of pain
- Sensations felt
- Previous injury

OBSERVATION is accomplished by visually inspecting the injured area for swelling (edema), discoloration (ecchymosis), deformity, and other signs of trauma.
- Swelling
- Ecchymosis (discoloration)
- Deformity
- Other signs of trauma

PALPATION begins when you evaluate the athlete's neurovascular status by checking circulatory and neurological functions. The next step is to palpate the site of injury - check for tenderness and deformity.
- Evaluate neurovascular status
- Palpate injury site
- Compare bilaterally

Then **STRESS** can begin. REMEMBER—When palpating and performing assessment tests, always compare bilaterally by examining the uninvolved extremity first. Perform assessment tests to

13

evaluate joint stability, inflammatory conditions, and to determine range of motion and strength.
• Perform assessment tests
• Evaluate joint stability
• Inflammatory conditions
• Determine range of motion and strength

Emergency Evaluation of the Unconscious Athlete

There are two major considerations in emergency evaluations: First, control of life threatening conditions, and second, management of non-life threatening injuries.

Primary Emergency Evaluation:
• Check to make sure the scene is safe for you to assist and call 911
• Check for open airway
• Check for abnormal or arrested breathing
• Check for abnormal or arrested pulse
• Check for excessive external bleeding
• Check for indicators of internal bleeding
• Check for shock
• Check for responsiveness (level of consciousness)

Secondary Emergency Evaluation:
• Check for head injury
• Check for spinal injury
• Check for dislocations and fractures
• Check for skin wounds

Treatment of Injuries (P.R.I.C.E.S.)

P: Protection: Once an injury has occurred, protect that injury from further damage. Never allow a bad injury to become worse. That may involve splinting the area, or just removing the athlete from participation.

R: Rest - Once an injury has occurred and the evaluation and first aid treatments are completed, rest the injury for at least a 24-hour period. The length of rest is dependent on the severity of the injury, therefore rest could easily be longer than 24 hours. Remove the athlete from competition and evaluate the injury.

I: Ice - Apply cold to the injured area. This will control bleeding and the associated swelling. This can be performed in one of two ways that are equally effective:
• Ice Packs: This should be done using plastic bags filled with ice covered with a wet towel This treatment should be done for 20 minutes, 6 to 8 times a day.
• Ice Immersion Bath: This should be done using a bath tub or large basin with a water temperature of between 50 - 60 degrees for 10 minutes, 6 to 8 times a day.
Note: Persons with any known circulation problems must avoid ice. If any problems arise, consult a physician.

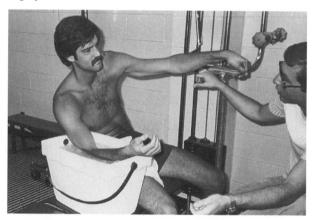

C: Compression: Utilize a compression (elastic) wrap to control swelling at the injured site. Begin the wrap distally (farthest from the heart) to the injury and spiral the wrap toward the heart. Note: Compression wraps should not be removed unless circulation or nerve function is interfered with. Things to look for:
• Extremities turning blue or pink.
• Numbness and tingling of extremities.
• Increased pain.
• Remove the wrap while sleeping.
• Remove the wrap every 4 hours for 15 minutes to allow the pressure to return to normal.

E: Elevation: Keep the injured body part elevated higher than the heart. This will allow gravity to keep excessive blood and associated swelling out of the injured area.

S: Support: Various techniques can be used to support an injury. If necessary, place the injured athlete on crutches for a lower extremity injury or use a sling for an upper extremity injury. This external support will allow the injury to be managed with better control.

First Aid and Emergency Care

The athletic trainer should follow the guidelines as established by the American Red Cross or the American Heart Association when giving first aid and emergency care. These national organizations have established protocols that will give the student athletic trainer the necessary guidance in this area.

The roles of the person applying first aid include prevention of further injury, reducing pain and stabilizing the injury. Athletic trainers and coaches can use their knowledge of the healing process so that recovery from athletic injuries is not delayed. Athletic trainers have found that if the athlete is untreated during the inflammation process, recovery will take longer than if the injury is aggressively treated. This is because proper first aid assists the body in protecting the area of injury and reduces the risk of further complications.

Extremity Splinting:

Fracture: *Any break in continuity of a bone*

Dislocation: *Displacement of the bone ends which form a joint*

Open: *Bone ends have broken through the skin or there is a wound which extends to the fracture site.*

Closed: *The skin has not been broken*

Signs: *Primary: Pain, tenderness, deformity, swelling*

Others: *Crepitus (grating), discoloration, loss of use, exposed fragments*

General Rules: All fractures should be "splinted as they lie," before transport. Long-bone fractures may be straightened with mild traction (which must then be maintained until splinted), but never attempt to straighten fractures or dislocations involving the spine or joints. To properly immobilize fractures, joints below and above the injury must be immobilized.

Emergency Equipment

A number of different types and styles of equipment, available for the athletic trainer, exist in the area of splinting. These range from inexpensive to quite costly, but they are all intended to do the same job - protect the injury from further damage. The following is a list of some commercially available splints.

Types of Splints:

• **Fixation Splints:** Most common and adaptable splint utilized. (Example: boards, wire, ladder, pillow, blankets)

• **Pneumatic** (air) Splints: Easy to apply and best suited for nondisplaced fractures, but not appropriate for dislocations.

• **Vacuum Splints:** Appropriate for dislocations or displaced fractures and adaptable to any limb angulation.

• **Traction Splints:** Used for long bone fracture, as in femur, and to prevent overriding of bones. Must have training in application of this splint. Used mostly in motor vehicle accidents. Example: Hair Traction Splint.

Vacuum Splint Application

Immobilization is the principle emergency procedure for fractures and dislocations. Proper immobilizations should prevent movement at the injury site and adjacent joints.

Advantages: Vacuum splints are best used in displaced fracture or joint dislocations. This splint is adaptable to any limb angulation.

Disadvantages: Vacuum splints are expensive. The splint can also develop a hole which prevents it from hardening and makes it ineffective.

Application: When using a vacuum splint one or two athletic trainer(s) should follow these steps.

• Inspection of the extremity for open wounds, deformity, swelling, and ecchymosis.

• Check **Pulse, Motor, Sensation (PMS) and capillary refill** at point below (distal) to the site of injury.

• Cover all wounds with a dry sterile dressing before applying a splint. Notify the receiving hospital of all open wounds.

• Do not move the athlete before splinting extremity injuries unless there is an immediate hazard to the athlete or yourself.

• Select proper splint. Length and size should cover above and below the injury site.

• Place splint beside the injured extremity, then smooth out the contents of the splint. The larger end of splint should be placed proximal to the injury.

• When applying the splint, use your hands to minimize movement. Also, support the injury above and below when applying the splint on the extremity. For stabilization purposes, apply a gentle traction to the limb.

• Secure splint with velcro straps, making a snug fit around the extremity while forming the splint to it.

• Remove air from the splint utilizing the vacuum splint hand pump. Splinting is achieved when a hard, rigid conforming brace completely immobilizes the injury.

• Again, check **Pulse, Motor, Sensation (PMS), and capillary refill** at a point distal to the site of injury.

• Ice can be applied over the vacuum splint and the injury can be X-rayed through the splint.

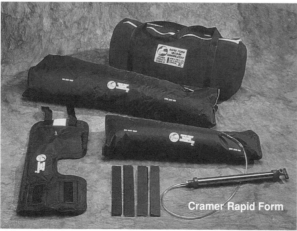
Cramer Rapid Form

Air Splint Application

The most commonly used formable or soft splint is the precontoured, inflatable, clear plastic air splint. These splints are available in a variety of sizes and shapes, with or without a zipper that runs the length of the splint.

Advantages: An air splint is comfortable for the patient, provides uniform contact, and applies firm pressure to a bleeding wound. These splints are commonly used in injuries that occur below the elbow or knee.

Disadvantages: Pressure of the air in splint will vary during weather changes (warm to cold to warm), and altitude changes. The zipper can stick, clog with dirt, or freeze. Plastic will be prone to stick to hot, perspiring skin, making application difficult. This type of splint does not allow the athletic trainer to check for sensory or motor movement, nor checking for associated pulse.

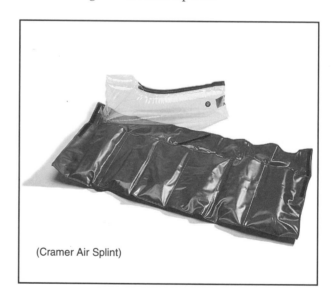
(Cramer Air Splint)

Application: When using a nonzippered or partially zippered type of air splint, the athletic trainer(s) should follow these steps:

• Inspect the limb for open wounds, deformity, swelling, and ecchymosis.

• Check **Pulse, Motor, Sensation (PMS) and capillary refill** of the injured site distal to the injury.

• Cover all open wounds with a dry sterile dressing before applying a splint. Notify the hospital of open wounds.

• First Athletic Trainer: Place your arm through the splint. Once your hand is extended beyond the splint, grasp the hand or foot of the injured limb.

• Second Athletic Trainer: Support the patient's injured limb until splinting is accomplished.

• First Athletic Trainer: Apply gentle traction to the hand or foot while sliding the splint onto the injured limb. The hand or foot of the injured limb should always be included in the splint.

• Inflate the splint by mouth, test for pressure by compressing the walls with a firm pinch between thumb and index finger. Splint should compress 1/2 to 1 inch.

• Again, check **Pulse, Motor, Sensation (PMS), and capillary refill** of the injured site distal to the injury.

• If circulation and/or neurological sensation is diminished, remove air from splint.

• Stabilize splint technique to body. For upper extremity injuries, swathe the splint to the body. Use long spine board for a lower extremity injury.

Long Spine Board/Logroll

The athlete with a head or neck injury (or unknown trauma) who is unconscious or exhibits motor weakness, paralysis, or decreased sensory function in one or more extremities should be handled definitively and carefully.

Application: When logrolling an athlete onto a long spine board, 4 or more athletic trainers or trained personnel are needed to perform the following emergency splinting.

• Monitor the vital signs; perform CPR if necessary. In a sport where a helmet and facemask are used, this protective equipment may impair access to the airway. The helmet should never be removed when dealing with a cervical injury, but the facemask or facemask clips may be cut with a Trainer's Angel. Always practice this procedure before an emergency occurs.

First Athletic Trainer: Apply and maintain cervical traction.

Second Athletic Trainer: Apply a cervical collar.

• First Athletic Trainer: Maintain inline traction.

• Second Athletic Trainer: Position at shoulders.

• Third Athletic Trainer: Position at hip and knee.

• Fourth Athletic Trainer: Position spine board behind injured athlete.

• On the command of the First Athletic Trainer, logroll injured athlete toward the athletic trainers while spineboard is slid under the injured athlete.

• Center injured athlete on long spine board.

• Pad any void between injured athlete and spine board.

• Secure head to long spine board by connecting a strip of tape from one side of the board across the forehead to the opposite side. A second strip is applied over the chin.

• Secure body to long spine board with strips of tape or buckles at shoulder, hip and knees.

• Secure the feet and arms to board.

• Check **Pulse, Motor, Sensation (PMS), and capillary refill** of the extremities.

• Remove front of cervical collar. Continue to monitor the vital signs.

Emergency Transportation Procedures

There are two points to consider in the area of transportation. The first is the availability of emergency ambulance service and the second is the severity of the injury. The student athletic trainer, staff athletic trainer, or coach should never transport an athlete in a private vehicle.

First Point: Availability of Emergency Ambulance Service: If there are services to your athletic competition, you should utilize those services. These people are skilled, practiced professionals who routinely provide advanced medical care and transport injured patients.

Second Point: Severity of Injury: Those injuries that are life threatening should be handled by Emergency Medical Technicians (EMTs). These professionals have the proper equipment and training to prepare athletes for transportation and vehicles equipped for safe and speedy transport. Those whose injuries are non-life threatening do not need to be transported in an emergency fashion, therefore the student athletic trainer can arrange for proper transportation of the athlete by either those adults in charge or by the parents/guardians.

Chapter 2 - Review Questions

Completion:

1. Upon arrival on the scene of an injury, the athletic trainer must first _____ the injured athlete.

2. When palpating and performing assessment tests, always compare _____ by examining the uninvolved extremity first.

3. The athletic trainer should not place his or her hands on an injured athlete until they have reached the _____ portion of HOPS.

4. List the recommended treatment time for an ice bag: _____.

5. Compression should be accomplished by using an _____ wrap.

6. Athletic trainers have discussed that if an athlete is left _____ during the inflammation process, recovery time will take _____.

7. A _____ splint should be used for long bone fractures.

8. Transportation of an injured athlete should never be performed by a student athletic trainer in a _____ _____.

Short Answer:

1. What is the first step in the injury process?

2. What is one of the primary function of an athletic trainer?

3. Why are assessment tests performed?

4. What is included in a secondary emergency evaluation?

5. What are the roles of a person applying first aid?

6. How should a fracture be properly immobilized?

7. What words do the letters H.O.P.S. represent?
   -
   -
   -
   -

8. What are the two major considerations in emergency evaluation?
   -
   -

9. What do the letters P.R.I.C.E.S. represent?
   -
   -
   -
   -
   -
   -

10. What are two equally effective procedures for applying cold to an injured area?
    -
    -

11. What are two advantages of an air splint?
    -
    -

12 What are the four different types of splints?
   -
   -
   -
   -

13. What are two important points to consider in the area of emergency transportation?
    -
    -

NOTES

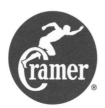

Chapter 3
Injuries And The Healing Process

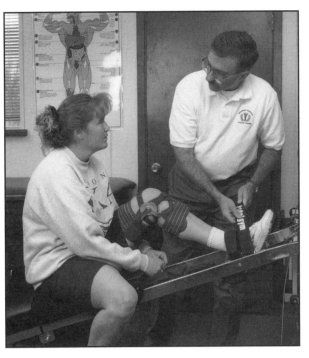

Educational Objectives

The learner should, at the completion of the chapter, be able to perform the following:

- Understand the inflammation process in healing of athletic injuries.
- Recognize the vital signs.
- Understand the treatment protocol of cold versus heat application.
- Distinguish between acute and chronic injury management.
- Identify the principles of physical rehabilitation and range of motion.
- Identify the more common musculoskeletal disorders encountered in athletic training.

Successful management of athletic injuries requires an understanding of what happens within the body in response to an injury. An awareness of how healing subsequently occurs is also required. With this understanding and awareness, the student athletic trainer can do more than take a textbook approach to first aid and follow-up treatments. Treatments can be individually structured to each athlete and to the body part injured. In this chapter, basic principles of healing will be discussed. The student athletic trainer will then be able to apply these principles to each of the anatomical sections covered in the following chapters. A complete understanding of this chapter is necessary before advancing to further chapters.

The Inflammation Process

When an athletic injury occurs, whether it is a strain, sprain, contusion, or open wound, the body immediately begins a process that eventually results in healing. This process is known as inflammation. In an acute injury, such as a muscle strain or ligament sprain, tissue is torn, capillaries are damaged, and cells die because of the interference in the blood and oxygen supply.

In response, the body reacts by sending specialized cells into the injury area in an attempt to limit damage and to begin healing. Among the functions of these cells is the initiation of blood clotting. In an attempt to limit the size of the damaged area, the body also reacts by contracting muscles in the injured area. This involuntary muscle spasm splints the area to restrict further movement and also reduces the local blood flow.

In acute injuries, the trauma and the body's reaction to the trauma result in **pain, swelling, and redness, heat and loss of function**. The pain is caused by increased pressure on nerve endings from internal hemorrhage and from the cellular response to lack of oxygen. **Swelling**, or edema, is caused by the accumulation of fluids in the damaged area. Hemorrhage, lymph fluid, and synovial fluid contribute to the swelling, increasing pressure on nerve endings. Gravity could also increase swelling if the limb is not elevated. **Redness** and a feeling of warmth occur once the healing process begins. The redness is due to the increased blood supply as the body attempts to provide the injury site with nutrients for repair.

When referring to an athletic injury, removal of unwanted items from the injured area precedes rebuilding. All the fluids and dead cells that have resulted in swelling must be removed from the injury site by the circulatory and lymphatic systems before oxygen and nutrient-supplying capillaries can be formed to assist repair. Removing the waste products and allowing oxygen and other nutrients to get to the damaged area will create a good environment for the formation of replacement tissue. This tissue is, in turn, gradually replaced by more specialized tissue, such as tendons.

Vital Signs

When evaluating an injured athlete, it is essential that the athletic trainer have a sound understanding of how to check the athlete's vital signs and what the standard values for the vital signs are. By knowing what the normal values are, the athletic trainer will be able to distinguish when an athlete's vital signs are abnormal. These would be evaluated in the primary survey of an emergency evaluation and, if necessary, are monitored throughout the entire evaluation and initial treatment.

Pulse

Adult 60-80/minute, Child 80-100/minute

Rapid but weak pulse could indicate shock, bleeding, diabetic coma, and/or heat exhaustion. A rapid and strong pulse typically indicates heat stroke and/or severe fright. A strong but slow pulse usually indicates a skull fracture and/or stroke. No pulse indicates cardiac arrest and/or death.

Respiration

Adult 12/minute, Child 20-25/minute

Breathing that is shallow usually indicates shock. Irregular or gasping breath could be cardiac related. Frothy blood from the mouth typically indicates a chest fracture (rib fracture).

Temperature

Oral 98.6 F, Rectal 99.6 F, Axillary 97.6 F

Hot, dry skin usually indicates disease, infection, and/or over-exposure to environmental heat. Typically, cool, clammy skin is an indicator of trauma, shock, and/or heat exhaustion. Overexposure to cold is displayed by cool, dry skin.

Skin Color

Red skin indicates heat stroke, diabetic coma, and/or high blood pressure. White (pale) skin means that the individual has insufficient circulation, shock, fright, hemorrhage, heat exhaustion, and/or insulin shock. Blue (cyanotic) skin indicates circulated blood is poorly oxygenated. The non-white athlete will still exhibit a paling of the skin, but you need to examine the inner lip and gum area. The same holds true for red and flushed, look at the lip and gum area.

Pupils

Constricted—sunlight, Dilated—dark room

In traumatic situations, pupils that are constricted usually indicate injury to the central nervous system and/or intake of a depressant drug. Dilated pupils (one or both eyes) could address head injury, shock, heat stroke, hemorrhage, and intake of a stimulant drug. When pupils fail to accommodate to light this could mean brain injury, intake of alcohol, or drug poisoning.

State Of Consciousness

When evaluating an individual's state of consciousness: awareness, memory, and response to commands are three important items to review.

Movement

Movement is classified in these basic aspects: active, passive, assistive, and resistive.

Abnormal Nerve Stimulation

When evaluating nerve stimulation, always check for motor (movement) and sensory (feeling) to determine if the affected area has nerve damage.

Blood Pressure

When the heart contracts, systolic pressure can be determined; as the heart relaxes, diastolic pressure can be found. Normal blood pressure in healthy adults is usually 120/80 (systolic/diastolic).

Treatment Protocols: Ice vs. Heat

When treating athletic injuries, selection of ice or heat application is critical. In most situations, ice should be used for the first 48 hours. At that time, re-evaluate the injury and determine if pain, swelling and redness are present. If they exist, continue the use of ice. If not, the philosophy of the medical staff will indicate when to use ice or heat. Listed below is a brief outline of types of ice and heat applications.

Application Of Ice

The basic physiological changes that occur through the use of ice on an injury include:
• Reduces swelling and inflammation
• Reduces blood flow to the injury site
• Reduces pain at the injury site

Cold Packs

Cold packs can be used for initial first aid or follow-up treatments. After placing crushed ice in a plastic bag, place a wet towel between the ice pack and affected body part and apply for a ten- to fifteen- minute period. This is the most economical way. Because of the danger of frostbite, the ice pack should not be applied directly to the skin. Also, the cold pack should be placed on the injury, not under the body where pressure can magnify possible damaging effects such as blistering or burning. Over a period of time, reusable cold packs may be more convenient than ice. While both the reusable cold pack and ice require pre-freezing, with the cold pack there is no mess as will be experienced with melting ice. Instant cold packs are also available for times when pre-frozen packs are not practical, but these are expensive and chemical burns can result if a leak occurs in the container.

Ice Massage

The technique of rubbing ice over an injured area is called ice massage. This treatment is applied, by the athletic trainer or athlete, directly to the skin. A paper or insulated cup is filled with water, then frozen. The cup is gradually peeled back as the athlete massages the injury site and the ice melts.

The treatment should last from 5-10 minutes depending on the depth and severity of the injury. To prevent skin damage move the ice cup continuously with a circular or back-and-forth motion. Ice massage should be avoided over bony areas.

Ice Water Immersion

This technique is used by immersing the injured extremity in cool water. Water temperature in a bucket or whirlpool tank should be 45-55 degrees. The injured part is kept in the cool water for five to ten minutes. With physician approval, the injured athlete then performs rehabilitation movements.

Cold Whirlpool

The whirlpool bath is a method for cold and warm water immersion. Duration of the treatment is usually 10 minutes and the temperature usually ranges from 50 to 60 degrees. The whirlpool offers a massaging effect.

Cold Spray

In certain situations, the use of cold sprays can be beneficial. Using caution, apply the spray to the affected area for no longer than 10 SECONDS. Since damage to the skin can occur, read the instructions prior to application. The application of cold spray to an injury will assist in reducing pain and swelling. Another name for cold spray is ethyl chloride. Because this technique only cools the surface, it is not nearly as effective as cold treatments.

Application Of Heat

The basic physiological changes that occur through the use of heat on an injury includes:
• Increased blood flow to the injured area
• Reduced muscle stiffness
• Muscular relaxation

Hot Packs

Pre-heated commercial hot packs are an efficient way to apply moist heat. Towels are used to insulate the pack and protect the skin from burning. Towels soaked in very hot water have the same effect as hot packs during the period of follow-up treatments, provided that proper insulation is placed between the skin and what could be damaging heat.

Hot Whirlpool

Also used for cold water immersion, the whirlpool bath is a popular method for warm water immersion. Used as a follow-up treatment, the disadvantages of whirlpool treatment include placing the injured part in a non-elevated, dependent position. Also, the equipment must be thoroughly cleaned daily to prevent the spread of disease. Duration of the treatment and temperature depend on the area of the body to be treated. Buckets of warm water can provide the same water-immersion effect as whirlpools. However, the whirlpool also offers a massaging effect.

Application Of Ice and Heat
Contrast Bath

The contrast bath is a follow-up treatment that combines hot and cold water immersion. Many types of injuries that have an increased amount of swelling seem to respond to the alternating of cold and heat. This type of treatment provides a pumping action, which assists in the removal of waste products caused by swelling.

Other Therapeutic Techniques
Exercise

Too often, EXERCISE is overlooked as a treatment. The movement of the body by the muscles increases circulation at a deeper level than the modalities that have been discussed. Exercise is used to maintain or increase strength and regain lost range of motion in order to assist in the healing process.

Massage

Because the friction of massage increases the temperature of the tissues and, therefore, increases local circulation, massage can be considered a heat treatment. Massage is used as a follow-up treatment for many injuries, especially muscle injuries. Besides increasing temperature, a massage can help to relax a muscle spasm in injured muscles. As with other

heat treatments, massage started too soon after an injury can restart internal bleeding. Additionally, massage is often used as an adjunct to stretching and warm-up exercises in many sports.

Counterirritants

Counterirritants are substances which, when applied to the skin, cause an irritation or reaction. This reaction can produce a sensation that is stronger than the sensation of minor pain. Long used by athletes, analgesic balms irritate the skin to provide a perception of warmth, which can help relax tight, aching muscles. Penetration of these analgesics is minimal. Their advantages include ease of application and availability. By covering the analgesic balm with a plastic-backed compress roll, the athletic trainer creates an analgesic pack. The pack can provide relief and a feeling of warmth to an athlete for hours. The compress roll also protects the clothes from staining. Some counterirritants can also provide a cooling sensation. Care should be taken not to apply counterirritants to an open or scabbed over wound.

Electrical Modalities

Various electrical modalities are used to decrease pain, swelling, and muscle spasm. Below is a brief list of commonly utilized modalities:
- Electrical Stimulating Currents
- Ultrasound
- Shortwave and Microwave Diathermy
- Ultraviolet Therapy
- Low-power Lasers

Acute vs Chronic Management
Acute Injuries

As with all injuries, the acute injury is handled by using the PRICES protocol. This includes the following components:

P: Protection - Protect the injury from further damage. Never allow a bad injury to become worse. This may include splinting the area, or just removing the athlete from participation.

R: Rest - Remove the athlete from participation and evaluate the injury.

I: Ice - Apply cold to the injured area. This will control internal bleeding and the associated swelling.

C: Compression - Utilize a compression (elastic) wrap to control swelling to the injured site. Begin the wrap distally to the injury and spiral the wrap toward the heart.

E: Elevation - Keep the injured body part elevated above the level of the heart. This will allow gravity to keep excess blood out of the area.

S: Support - If necessary, place the injured athlete on crutches for a lower extremity injury or use a sling for an upper extremity injury. This external support will allow for the injury to be managed with better control.

Chronic Injuries

The management of chronic injuries is characterized by the continued use of cold, but is coupled with exercise, modality use, and a variety of heat/cold combination treatments.

Principles of Physical Rehabilitation

The goal of a sound rehabilitation program is to return the injured athlete to pre-injury levels of strength, power, endurance, flexibility, and confidence as quickly and safely as possible. A rehabilitation program is concerned not with just the injured body part, but also with preventing deconditioning of the rest of the body. If the athlete returns to activity without undergoing physical rehabilitation, that athlete could easily become re-injured. Typically, the injured athlete is an exceptional patient, motivated to get well and to overcome the injury. Of course, some athletes are more motivated than others. Some athletes will have to be pushed and encouraged daily during their rehabilitation, while others will need to be restrained from trying to rush their recovery. Open communication between the coach and physician regarding the athlete's progress is critical.

In an ideal situation, the physician will work with the athletic trainer or the coach on setting up an individualized rehabilitation program. After approving initiation of the program, there are two principles that must be observed: pain should be avoided, and the athlete must be encouraged to follow the program. Pain can be avoided by total rest. However, an aggressive rehabilitation program will require a particular exercise program by the athlete at a level slightly less than what causes pain. Daily adherence to a rehabilitation program benefits the athlete in several ways. First, the athlete stays in the habit of working out. Also, daily exercise will result in tangible results; missing even one day will result in a loss of strength or conditioning. Psychologically, the athlete will feel better about himself/herself if allowed to participate in his/her own recovery, rather than watching practice. The athletic trainer should set specific times each day for the athlete to work on his or her rehabilitation program.

A comprehensive rehabilitation program is critical to the injured athlete. In designing this program, the following five phases of physical rehabilitation need to be addressed. Phases of rehabilitation are:
- Post-surgical/acute injury
- Early exercise
- Intermediate exercise
- Advanced exercise
- Initial sports reentry

An athlete will move through all five phases of the rehabilitation program on the way to complete recovery. The athletic trainer must keep in mind that each athlete and each injury is different. Various rates of recovery should be expected.

Basic Principles of Physical Rehabilitation

Physical rehabilitation is a major area of concern to health professionals participating in a sports medicine environment. Athletic competition requires that rehabilitation be aggressive. In most cases, the goal is to return the athlete to activity at the pre-injury level as quickly and as safely as possible. While rehabilitation uses prescribed exercise to return individuals to activity, rehabilitation techniques can also help prevent injuries. In planning a physical rehabilitation program, the athletic trainer deals with these several components:

- Decrease pain and effusion
- Decrease the inflammatory response to trauma
- Return of full, pain-free active range of motion
- Return of full muscular strength, power, and endurance
- Return to full asymptomatic functional activities at the pre-injury level

During the physical rehabilitation process, be aware of the effects of immobilization:
- Muscle atrophy
- Arthrofibrosis
- Articular cartilage softening
- Decrease in ligament strength
- Increase in uptake of bone

There are three basic components of any physical rehabilitation program:
- Therapeutic exercise
- Therapeutic modalities
- Athlete education

When determining the purpose of the exercise always consider the following:
- Joint range of motion

- Muscle flexibility
- Muscular strength, power and endurance
- Balance, proprioception, and kinesthetic awareness
- Cardiovascular fitness (total body conditioning)

Progressive resistive exercises may be used to increase muscular strength, power, and endurance. These exercises may be:
- Isometric
- Isotonic
- Isokinetic

The seven components an athletic trainer is concerned with in planning a physical rehabilitation program are:
- Joint motion
- Muscular strength
- Muscular power
- Muscular endurance
- Muscular flexibility
- Proprioception
- Cardiovascular performance

Range Of Motion

Assessing joint range of motion is critical in evaluating injuries. The athletic trainer should gain experience in using a goniometer. Listed below is a brief outline of ranges of motion for anatomical joints. Use this as a guideline in assessing movement.

Ankle
Dorsiflexion - 45 degrees
Plantarflexion - 20 degrees
Inversion - 40 degrees
Eversion - 20 degrees

Knee
Flexion - 140 degrees
Extension - 0 degree

Hip
Flexion - 125 degrees
Extension - 10 degrees
Adduction - 40 degrees
Abduction - 45 degrees

Shoulder
Flexion - 180 degrees
Extension - 45 degrees
Adduction - 40 degrees
Abduction - 180 degrees
Internal Rotation - 90 degrees
External Rotation - 90 degrees

Elbow
Flexion - 140 degrees
Extension - 0 degrees

Forearm
Pronation - 80 degrees
Supination - 85 degrees

Wrist
Flexion - 80 degrees
Extension - 70 degrees
Adduction - 45 degrees
Abduction - 20 degrees

General Musculoskeletal Disorders

When treating injuries, an understanding of specific disorders is important. Please review these disorders and discuss the specific treatment required with your athletic trainer and team physician.

Arthritis—*inflammation of a joint*
Atrophy— *the wasting away of a normally developed organ or tissue due to degeneration of cells.*

Bursitis—*inflammation of a bursa*

Contracture— *fibrosis of muscle tissue producing shrinkage and shortening of the muscle without generating any strength.*

Contusion—*a bruise; an injury usually caused by a blow in which the skin is not broken*

Dislocation—*the displacement of one or more bones or a joint, or of any organ from the original position*

Epicondylitis—*inflammation of the epicondyle and the tissues adjoining the epicondyle to the humerus (Pitcher's elbow-medial epicondyle, Tennis elbow-lateral epicondyle)*

Fascitis—*inflammation of a fascia*

Myositis—*inflammation of muscle tissue*

Myositis Ossificans—*inflammation of muscle, with formation of bone*

Sprain—*a wrenching of a joint, producing a stretching or laceration of the ligaments*

Strain—*excessive stretching or overuse of a part, as tendon/muscle*

Subluxation—*a partial or incomplete dislocation*

Synovitis—*inflammation of the synovial membrane*

Tendinitis—*inflammation to the tendon*

Tenosynovitis—*inflammation of tendon sheath*

Chapter 3 - Review Questions

Completion:

1. The body's reaction to trauma are _____, _____, and _____.

2. Redness and a feeling of warmth around an injury are signs of an increase of _____ to that body part.

3. Normal pulse readings for adults are _____, and children are _____.

4. Normal blood pressure of a healthy adult is ____/____.

5. Ice is used initially on an injury to control _____, _____, and _____.

6. Types of heat application are _____ and _____.

7. Chronic injuries are treated with _____, _____, _____, and _____ treatments.

8. Range of motion of a joint can be measured by using a _____.

9. Specialized cells initiate blood _____ .

10. All the fluids and dead cells that have resulted in swelling must be removed from the injury site by the _____ and _____ systems.

11. Constricted pupils are a sign of CNS _____ drug use.

12. A rehabilitation program should be focused not only on the injured body part, but also on preventing _____ of the rest of the body.

Short Answer:

1. What are the three types of progressive resistance exercises?
*
*
*

2. What five phases of physical rehabilitation need to be included in a comprehensive rehabilitation program?
*
*
*
*
*

3. List three physiological factors associated with ice:

•

•

•

4. List three physiological factors associated with heat:

•

•

•

5. Why is gaining normal range of motion important?

6. Explain the difference between arthritis and bursitis.

7. Explain the difference between a sprain and a strain.

NOTES

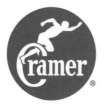

Chapter 4
Biohazardous Protocols

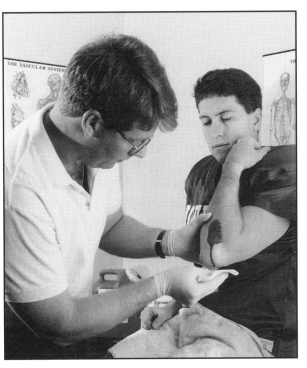

Educational Objectives

The learner should, at the completion of the chapter, be able to perform the following:

- Recognize the classification and management of wounds.
- Understand the need to comply with Occupational Safety and Health Administration (OSHA) guidelines.
- Identify the prevalent bloodborne pathogens commonly seen in athletic training.
- Understand the protocol in waste management.
- Recognize the National High School Federation rules as they relate to biohazardous materials.

Classification and Management of Wounds

Wounds involve a compromise to the integumentary (skin) system. There are differences in types of wounds centering around the method that breaks the skin. The principle classifications of wounds include:

- Abrasions
- Avulsions
- Incisions
- Lacerations
- Punctures

The following segment describes the different types of wounds, the initial care, and follow-up care for each.

Wound Management

Abrasions

Description: Outer layers of skin are damaged from being scraped on a hard surface. Bleeding is limited due to the rupture of small veins and capillaries. Infection could occur if dirt is ground into the torn tissues.

Initial Care: Put on latex gloves. Cleanse abraded area with Cinder Suds and sterile gauze pads. Scrub dirt away from the wound. Apply povidone-iodine solution over the injury. Place Strawberry Ointment on an adhesive bandage strip and apply to keep the wound moist.

Follow-up Care: Change dressing daily. Watch for infection. Keep the wound moist with Strawberry Ointment so that a scab does not form. A scab will keep getting knocked off and will create more bleeding as well as a larger scab.

Avulsions

Description: A forcible separation or tearing of tissue from the body. Heavy and rapid bleeding ensues immediately.

Initial Care: Put on latex gloves. Clean around the wound with povidone-iodine solution. Do not wipe anything into the wound. Apply sterile gauze pad over the wound. Wrap the avulsed body part in a gauze pad. Place the covered, avulsed body part in cold container. Elevate the injured area higher than the heart and transport the injured athlete and the avulsed body part to a physician. The physician may be able to reattach the avulsed part. Tetanus toxoid injection may be needed.

Follow-up Care: Follow the physician's directions in changing dressings. Monitor any signs of infection.

Incision

Description: A sharp-cut wound caused by a sharp object such as glass or metal. Deep cuts will cause rapid and heavy bleeding; they may also damage muscles, tendons, and nerves.

Initial Care: Put on latex gloves. For superficial cuts, clean with Nitrotan and a gauze pad; place Bacitracin on a bandage strip and apply this bandage. For deep incisions, cleanse around the wound with povidone-iodine solution. Apply a gauze pad over the wound and wrap in place with tape and an elastic wrap for compression. Take athlete to a physician; a tetanus toxoid may be needed, as well as sutures.

Follow-up Care: Follow the physician's directions in changing the dressings. Watch for signs of infection. For superficial cuts that did not require physician intervention, be alert for signs of infection. Clean and change dressing regularly using the same initial care. At the first signs of infection, refer the athlete to a physician.

Laceration

Description: A jagged, irregular tear in the soft tissues.

Initial Care: Put on latex gloves. Use the same care as with incisions—superficial and deep.

Follow-up Care: Use the same follow-up care as with incisions.

Puncture

Description: A small hole in the tissues produced by an object (such as a nail) piercing the skin layers. External bleeding is limited; however, internal damage to organs may cause vast internal bleeding.

Initial Care: Clean around the wound with Nitrotan. Do not remove anything from the wound, but rather bandage it in place and refer to a physician. A tetanus toxoid may be needed.

Follow-up Care: Follow the physician's directions in changing dressing. Watch for signs of infection. Puncture wounds are more likely to become infected because they lack the external bleeding that will help flush out the contaminants of other types of wounds.

Occupational Safety and Health Administration (OSHA) Guidelines

Nearly two years after the OSHA regulations concerning exposure to bloodborne pathogens in the workplace were published, confusion and myths still abound. This concern is for two reasons.

First, it is clear most schools do not understand the scope of the standard because the vast majority are not in compliance. Unfortunately, the fact that a school or company does not fully understand the standard will not protect it from enforcement penalties should OSHA ever inspect your facility.

Second, while the risk of actual infection with a bloodborne disease is still relatively small, it is growing, especially from Hepatitis B. While the OSHA regulations are cumbersome and time consuming to follow, they should be effective in reducing the risk of infection even further and, therefore, will help stop the spread of bloodborne diseases.

It is estimated that there are 1.5 million people infected with the HIV virus, the majority of whom do not have visible symptoms of the disease. How many new cases develop each year is unknown, but the total number of known cases has grown from about 2,000 in 1976 to the current 1.5 million. The Center for Disease Control (CDC) estimates the total number of new Hepatitis B infections each year to be about 300,000.

In order to further everyone's understanding of the OSHA standard and some of its issues surrounding it, The First Aider, addressed some of the most frequently asked questions.

What is the OSHA bloodborne pathogens standard?

OSHA Regulation 1910.1030, Occupational Exposure to Bloodborne Pathogens, sets forth required procedures for protecting employees of any type of company, organization, institution against accidental exposure to bloodborne pathogens. This standard was first published in the Federal Register on December 6, 1991 and became effective March 6, 1992.

Is my school covered by this standard?

If your school has employees who, in the course of the work which has been assigned to them, can reasonably be expected to come into contact with human blood, certain body fluids, or infectious waste, it must comply with the provisions of OSHA 1910.1030.

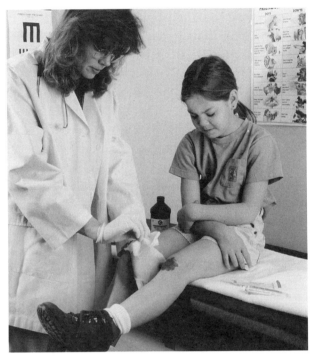

Adequate protection and protocols must be followed by all schools.

In a scholastic setting, who might be at risk of exposure?

The most obvious employees are athletic trainers, coaches, and school nurses who are first responders to athletic or other injuries. The basketball or wrestling coach dealing with a bloody nose or split lip is considered to be in the presence of infectious material. The athletic trainer treating a common abrasion makes his or her employer subject to the standard.

Less obvious are teachers providing first aid, the custodial personnel required to mop the gym floor or wrestling mat upon which blood has been spilled, and the laundry workers who must handle blood soaked uniforms. All of these employees are covered by the standard, and provided its protection.

Are game officials and referees considered employees?

Yes. As soon as a high school hires them to work a game or match, they are technically considered to be employees of the school and the protections spelled out in the standard must be provided to them.

What are the basic provisions of OSHA 1910.1030?

The bloodborne pathogens standard involves seven very precisely defined areas. They are:

1. Scope (identifies employees covered)
2. Exposure control plan (a written, site-specific plan outlining the steps to be taken to minimize employee exposure to bloodborne pathogens)
3. Methods of compliance (written procedures on how to control exposure)
4. Vaccinations and medical evaluations (outlines Hepatitis B vaccination requirements and post exposure medical evaluation and follow-up)
5. Information and training (explains requirements for communicating standard to employees)
6. Recordkeeping (defines records that must be kept)
7. Dates (provides schedule of implementation)

Can the NCAA, NAIA, National Federation or any other governing body issue rules which supersede the OSHA standard?

All have issued guidelines covering exposure to infectious substances. In general, these are designed to protect student athletes and do not address the total requirements of protecting employees. No guidelines supersede the OSHA standard.

If my school is in compliance with regulations of its governing body, is it in compliance with the OSHA Standard?

No. Unless the regulations of the organization are at least as comprehensive as OSHA 1910.1030 they would not be a substitute for them.

Can our teams remove blood from a player's uniform and be in compliance with the OSHA Standard?

There is nothing in the standard which specifically prohibits the removal of blood from uniforms. However, the standard does stipulate the only approved method of removing blood from a uniform is to put the uniform through a complete wash cycle with a commercial laundry detergent. Since the intent of the standard is to protect employees from exposure to bloodborne pathogens and employees such as referees, equipment managers, and laundry personnel could conceivably be exposed through an improperly disinfected uniform, OSHA would most likely discourage the practice of removing blood from uniforms with a chemical spot remover.

What about spraying a disinfectant on the blood spot?

This method is not approved as an effective means to disinfect a potentially contaminated uniform. Blood on uniforms is absorbed by thousands of threads made of additional thousands of microscopic fibers. The extent to which a disinfectant will kill viruses and tuberculosis bacilli under these circumstances has not been verified. Presently utilized CDC testing methods apply to hard, non-absorbent surfaces only.

(The above came from The First Aider, Winter 1994, Vol. 64, No. 2)

Bloodborne Pathogens

As athletic trainers, our primary concern is the health of our athletes. Unfortunately, we must now also be concerned for our own personal safety. In 1992, OSHA issued new regulations regarding health care workers and the handling of bloodborne pathogens (BBP).

The bloodborne pathogens of most concern are HIV and Hepatitis B. These BBPs are of special concern to the athletic trainer since it is common for the athletic trainer to come in contact with blood and other body fluids on a daily basis. It is possible we may be infected by the very athletes we are trying to help. This contamination is potentially lethal.

It is foolish for the athletic trainer to assume none of these athletes are contaminated. Therefore, we should know and practice proper preventive measures. Fortunately, OSHA has laid down basic guidelines for the health care professional.

Gloves

An athletic trainer can be exposed to BBPs in a variety of ways. The most obvious is caring for an

---

Waste Management

Preparing the 1:10 Bleach Solution:

1. In a spray bottle, add 1 ounce of bleach to 9 ounces of water. The bleach should be mixed with cool water. Warm or hot water deactivates the bleach's basic cleaning agent, "hypochlorite."
2. Label the bottle and store it so it is accessible only to those who are going to use it.
3. This solution mixture is good only one day. To be effective, the solution must be made daily.

Use of Bleach Cleaning Solution:

The following procedure is recommended to clean up body fluids:

1. After putting on gloves, absorb the fluids with paper towels.
2. Scrub the area with soap and water using a paper towel.
3. Rinse the area.
4. Saturate the area with bleach solution and allow to soak 20 minutes before absorbing it with another paper towel.
5. All soiled materials, including gloves, should be placed in the biohazard container.
6. Wash hands thoroughly after disposal of materials.

(The above came from The First Aider, Fall 1992, Vol. 62, No. 1)

athlete with some sort of bloody wound. Other situations would include serum fluid in blisters, vomitus with an ill athlete, and saliva in spittle.

Given these exposure opportunities, the athletic trainer should take proper precautions. First, wear latex gloves when working on athletes with exposed body fluids. The use of gloves provides a barrier between you and the wound or body fluid you are treating. Gloves should be worn at all times when evaluating an athlete, especially when the possibility of an undiscovered, open wound may exist.

When wearing latex gloves, there are some general guidelines an athletic trainer should follow. First, the protective value of the gloves diminishes after 10-15 minutes of wearing them. If gloves should tear, replace them immediately. When choosing gloves, an athletic trainer should select a size which fits his or her hands. After use, the gloves and all contaminated materials should be disposed of properly in a biohazard infectious waste container.

The next protection tip athletic trainers should follow is cleaning of the contaminated athletic training room. An effective preparation is a 1 to 10 bleach/water solution.

National High School Federation Rules

In March of 1994, the National Federation of State High School Associations adopted its nine point Communicable Disease Procedures. This document outlines the protocols that should be followed in the handling of bodily fluids. The nine points include:

- Stop bleeding and remove blood from uniforms
- Use precautions when handling body fluids
- Wash body surfaces exposed to body fluids
- Clean all surfaces and equipment before resuming play
- Properly dispose of sharps and body fluids
- Use artificial ventilation devices when performing CPR
- Support personnel must follow precautions if their skin is broken
- Proper cleaning and/or disposal of blood soaked towels
- Follow accepted guidelines for controlling bleeding

These guidelines are not identical to the OSHA guidelines or universal precautions. The safety of all people involved is the most important point to remember. Therefore, follow the guidelines that give you the most protection and safety.

In addition to establishing Communicable Disease Procedures, the NFSHSA also has specific rules on bleeding players. Those sports involved with specific rules include baseball, softball, basketball, field hockey, football, gymnastics, ice hockey, soccer, spirit (cheerleading), swimming & diving, track & field, volleyball, water polo, and wrestling. For more information, contact the NFSHSA regarding the specifics of each sport.

Chapter 4 - Review Questions

Completion:

1. Wounds effect the _____, also known as the integumentary system.

2. In all follow-up wound care, the athletic trainer should look for signs of _____.

3. All soiled material should be placed in a _____ _____.

4. A student athletic trainer should look for signs of _____ each day when changing wound dressings.

5. OSHA guidelines cover bloodborne pathogens such as _____ and _____.

6. Bleach should be mixed with _____ water.

7. Latex gloves provide a barrier between you and the wound or _____ _____.

8. The CDC estimates about _____ infections each year of Hepatitis B.

9. A _____ is when the outer layer of skin is scraped or scratched.

10. An incision is usually caused by a _____.

11. In a puncture wound, the object should _____ be removed.

12. Wounds should be cleaned with a disinfectant such as _____ or _____.

Short Answer:

1. List the five types of wounds mentioned in this chapter.
-
-
-
-
-

2. Name three of the nine Communicable Disease Procedures.
-
-
-

3. What is the difference between a laceration vs. avulsion?

4. Who might be at risk of exposure to blood borne pathogens?

5. What are the bloodborne pathogens that are of most concern in today's health care?

6. What solution is used to clean a contaminated athletic training room area?

7. How long does the bleach/water solution keep its effectiveness?

8. How do OSHA guidelines apply to laundry handlers?

9. List the initial care for an avulsion.

NOTES

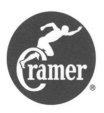

Chapter 5

Preventive And Supportive Techniques

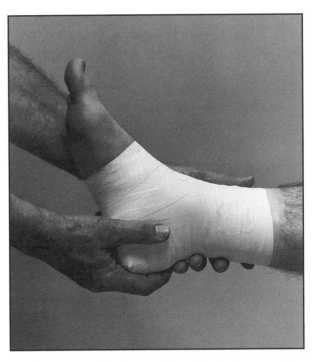

Educational Objectives

The learner should, at the completion of the chapter, be able to perform the following:

- Understand the principles of preventive techniques.
- Recognize the proper selection of supplies and equipment in this area.
- Identify the protocol in preparation of taping and/or wrapping.
- Identify the proper steps in the application and removal of taping techniques.
- Understand the guidelines for the application of elastic wraps.
- Recognize the precautions an athletic trainer must take in the application of preventive techniques.

Principles of Preventive Techniques

The primary purpose for the application of tape and/or elastic wrap is to provide additional support and stability for the affected body part. Through proper application, taping/wrapping techniques can be applied to shorten the angle of pull of muscles and decrease joint range of motion. Elastic wrap can be used for compression and/or support. Compression wraps are utilized in initial injury treatment protocol of protection, rest, ice, compression, elevation, and support (P.R.I.C.E.S.). In applying a compression wrap, use a spiral pattern, and beginning distal to the injury, wrap toward the heart. During athletic activities elastic wraps may also be utilized for support. Likewise, adhesive and elastic tapes can be utilized for both acute and chronic injuries. In instances when tape is applied over a joint, the purpose is to assist in the stabilization of the bones and necessary structures.

Furthermore, adhesive and/or elastic tape can be utilized to secure pads, braces, dressings, and/or elastic wraps.

While the basic principles of taping and wrapping are presented in this chapter, the learner should consult the textbook *The Comprehensive Manual for Taping and Wrapping Techniques* for full descriptions of taping application and removal.

Supplies and Equipment

In this chapter, the terminology for tape will either be adhesive tape or elastic tape. Adhesive tape is traditionally marketed as non-elastic, white tape. Elastic tape provides greater freedom of mobility to the affected body part. Both adhesive and elastic tapes are produced in a variety of widths. Elastic wrap is a woven fabric that also allows for expansion and contraction, in which either compression or supportive techniques can be utilized. This product typically is produced in widths of 2, 3, 4 and 6 inch, and length of normal or extra long.

In the preparation of some body parts, protection of the skin must be considered. In those situations, adhesive bandages, gauze underwrap, and/or grease pads should be applied. One of the most critical aspects of taping/wrapping techniques is the selection of proper supplies. Depending on the number and types of sports offered and frequency of injury, a variety of supplies should be made available. Purchasing supplies will depend on budget, philosophy of medical staff regarding taping/wrapping techniques, and type/frequency of injury.

Special consideration must be given to these additional factors: use of spray adherent, adhesive versus elastic tape, width of adhesive and elastic tape, and length and width of elastic wraps.

Preparation for Taping and Wrapping Procedures

In preparing the body for the application of tape and/or wrap, six items need to be considered.

• **Removal of hair:** The athlete should shave the body part where the technique will be applied. This will insure a good solid foundation for the tape and/or wrap and allow for easy removal of the tape as well as reduce irritation to the skin.

• **Clean the area:** Once the hair has been removed, make sure the skin is clean and free of moisture.

• **Special considerations:** Protection of the skin is important. Special care must be provided if the skin has any of the following conditions: allergies, infections, or open and closed wounds. Prior to the application of any taping/wrapping technique, consult a physician regarding the proper care of these medical conditions. With any of these conditions, the athletes must have proper pre-and post-activity care. It is preferred that medicated ointment and garment barrier adhesive bandages, gauze, underwrap, etc.) be placed on the skin. This will help prevent the skin from becoming more irritated. Since blisters are the most common problem, high friction areas need to be protected. Once a blister has developed, the area must be cleaned, dressed, and padded prior to the application of the taping technique.

• **Spray adherent:** The affected area that is to be supported by tape and/or wrap should be sprayed with an adherent. This will aid the adhesive quality of the application and thus provide stability to the supportive technique.

• **Skin lubricants:** In areas of high friction or sensitivity (i.e., Achilles tendon and top of the foot where the ankle flexes), a skin lubricant along with a heel and lace pad applied to the area will help reduce the possibility of irritation.

• **Underwrap:** This product can also be used in conjunction with lubricated heel and lace pads. This foam wrap should primarily be used in cases where the athlete is allergic to tape and to hold heel and lace pads in place at high friction areas. When underwrap is used to cover the entire taping area, stability of the taping technique may be compromised.

Application and Removal of Taping Techniques

Tearing adhesive tape

The adhesive tape is held firmly on each side of the point of the proposed tear line. With proper tension applied on the tape, the free end is pulled away at an angle so that the force crosses the lines of the fabric of the backcloth at a sharp angle. The tear then occurs sequentially through the backcloth. The more quickly and deftly this maneuver is done, the more evenly tape edges will be torn.

Some brands of elastic tape are extremely hard to tear by hand. It is recommended that those brands be cut with scissors to insure proper tape application and neatness.

Proper body positioning

Before beginning any taping procedure, have the athlete assume an anatomically correct and comfortable position so that they can maintain this position until the procedure is finished. Do not allow them to move around or "test" the technique before you have completed the procedure. Select a comfortable table height and position yourself in a good postural alignment to minimize strain and fatigue.

Removal of tape, adherent, and residue

Easy removal of adhesive and elastic tape is accomplished by using bandage scissors or a specially constructed tape cutter. A small amount of lubricant on the tip of the cutting device will allow the instrument to slip under the tape more readily, thus allowing removal of the tape with ease. Avoiding bony prominences, move the scissors or cutter along the natural channels or in areas of greatest soft tissue cushion. Once this has been completed, remove the tape from the skin in a constant and gradual manner. It is preferred that the tape be removed in the opposite direction from which it was applied. When pulling the tape from the skin at an angle of 180 degrees, care should be exercised to minimize removal of skin tissue and creation of skin irritation. It is recommended that pressure be applied to the skin (pull the skin away from the tape), which will reduce the possibility of skin irritation. The daily use of a tape remover is recommended to help keep the skin clean and to prevent skin irritations and/or infections. Tape remover and/or alcohol will aid in the removal of tape mass and adherent from the skin. Basic guidelines could include:

- Remove the tape immediately after its function has been served.
- Avoid irritating or tearing the skin.
- When using scissors or a tape cutter, avoid gouging the skin.
- Have the athlete gently massage the skin with a moisturizing skin massage lotion, especially if suffering from dry skin.
- Watch for signs of tape rash or an allergic reaction to the tape or tape adherent.

Proper skin care

It is advised that proper skin care be encouraged for those individuals who have tape applied to their skin. In these situations, a skin moisturizing cream may be used to prevent excessive dryness upon removal of the tape. In no instance should an athlete apply a skin moisturizer just prior to the application of any taping/wrapping technique. Such action will greatly reduce the required stabilizing effect of the tape job. If an individual has developed allergies, infections, or open or closed wounds, please consult a physician regarding the proper care of these medical conditions.

Guidelines for Applying Elastic Wraps

Elastic wraps can be made of cotton or polyester, and they come in various widths and lengths for specific purposes. The most common sizes are the 2-inch (for the hand, wrist and ankle), the 3-inch (for the elbow and knee) and the 4 or 6-inch (for the

thigh, groin and trunk). Standard length for elastic wraps is 5-yards, with double-length wraps often used in the 4- and 6-inch widths. Use the following guidelines when applying elastic wraps.

- The muscles of the body part to be wrapped should be contracted to prevent impaired circulation.
- Hold the loose end of the wrap on the body part and unroll the wrap from the bottom of the roll.
- Anchor the wrap with at least two turns around the body part.
- Keep even, uniform pressure on the wrap; excessive pressure can restrict circulation.
- Overlap each turn of the wrap by at least one-half its width to prevent pinching of the skin.
- Check for comfort and signs of impaired circulation.

For parts of the body that are difficult to provide compression, felt or foam pads can be cut to size and applied for additional compression. For example, a U-shaped pad held in place with an elastic wrap can provide extra compression for ankle sprains.

Precautions
Temperature of skin

Prior to applying any technique, the skin temperature should be normal. After any therapeutic treatment, it is advisable to allow adequate time to expire, which will allow the skin to return to its normal temperature. This reduces the chances of skin irritation.

Increasing risk

The safety of the athlete should be foremost in the mind of the person applying the support techniques. Because the improper application of tape and/or wrap could cause further injury to a body part, caution must be used in the application of any procedure. For all injured athletes, consultation with a physician is recommended. The application of tape should not be used to allow participation with any disabling conditions.

Chapter 5 - Review Questions

Completion:

1. Elastic tape has the ability to _____ and _____.

2. Athletes should not apply a _____ just prior to the application of any tape.

3. _____ are used in the initial treatment of acute injuries.

4. Proper skin temperature reduces the chances of _____ .

5. Taping and wrapping procedures are not a substitute for proper _____ .

6. The _____ should be consulted in case of immobilization.

Short Answer:

1. What is the primary purpose for tape or elastic wraps?

2. How is a compression wrap applied?

3. What is the terminology for tape?

4. In preparation of some body parts for applying tape, what would be applied for protection of the skin?

5. What is the importance of skin lubricants?

6. What is the proper body positioning for taping an athlete?

7. Why is the daily use of a tape remover recommended?

8. What are elastic wraps made of?

9. What can be used for body parts which are difficult to to provide compression?

10. What should the skin temperature be for applying any taping technique?

11. Why should caution be used in the application of any procedure?

12. What is the advantage to removing hair prior to taping?

13. What is the primary purpose for applying tape or an elastic wrap?

14. What are the six items to be considered before application of tape and/or wrap?
    *
    *
    *
    *
    *
    *

15. List three considerations to keep in mind when applying foam.
    *
    *
    *

NOTES

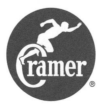

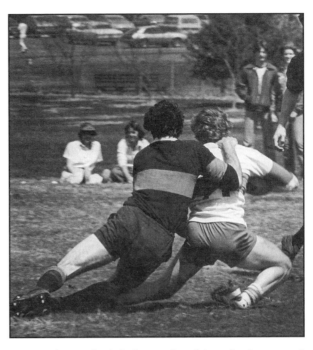

Chapter 6
The Foot, Ankle, and Lower Leg

Educational Objectives

The learner should, at the completion of the chapter, be able to perform the following:

- Understand the anatomy of the foot, ankle, and lower leg.
- Identify the components of an evaluation format.
- Recognize the common injuries associated with this part of the lower extremity.
- Understand the principles of rehabilitation for this part of the lower extremity.
- Understand the taping and wrapping techniques for this part of the lower extremity.
- Identify the NATA competencies for this region of the body.

Anatomy

The foot is the site of some of the most minor, yet irritating, conditions suffered by athletes. Examples of these conditions include blisters, calluses, athlete's foot, and ingrown toenails. Left untreated, these conditions can be just as disabling for an athlete as some of the more serious foot problems, such as heel bruises, arch strains, and fractures. The foot has stresses placed on it that exceed the demands placed on any other area of the body. This area stabilizes and supports the rest of the body while standing, walking, running, or jumping. Whether the impact with the ground is on the heel (as in jogging), the ball of the foot (as in running), or the toes (as in sprinting), the foot responds by absorbing several hundred pounds of force up to three times the body weight. Individually, the parts of the foot (bones, muscles, ligaments) are relatively weak. As a whole, however, the foot is strong enough to withstand most of the demands of athletics. The key to the foot's function is a set of

four arches, which help in absorbing the impact of walking, running, and jumping. The arches are called:

- Transverse arch
- Metatarsal arch
- Inner longitudinal arch
- Outer longitudinal arch

The feet contain about one-fourth of the total number of bones in the body. Each foot has 26 bones (7 tarsal bones, 5 metatarsal, and 14 phalanges) and 38 joints. The tarsal bones are the talus, calcaneus, navicular, cuboid, and the medial, intermediate, and lateral cuneiform bones. The mid foot region is made up of the 5 metatarsal bones. The toes have total 14 bones known as the phalanges.

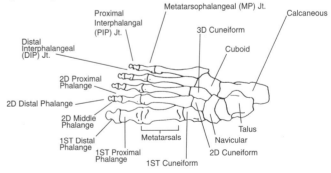

The Bones of the Foot

The ankle is the most commonly injured major joint in athletics. Fortunately, most injuries are minor ligament sprains. Knowledge of the ankle's anatomy, its mechanism of injury, first aid, wrapping, and taping are essential.

The ankle joint is formed by four bones: the tibia, fibula, talus, and calcaneus. The tibia and fibula are the two bones of the lower leg, while the talus and calcaneus are the two largest bones of the foot. Those large, bony prominences (malleoli) on either side of the ankle are the distal heads of the tibia (medially) and the fibula (laterally).

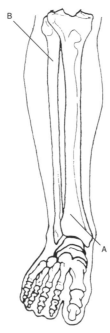

The bones of the lower leg are the tibia (A) and the fibula (B). Both of these bones are susceptible to stress fracures, often diagnosis and treatment are essential as continued stress will lead to a worsening of the fracture.

The tibia, which transmits the weight or force placed on the lower leg to the talus, is mounted almost directly on top of the talus and extends over its medial side. On the lateral side of the talus the fibula extends, forming the lateral malleolus and helping to stabilize the ankle joint. Because of this configuration of bones, the ankle is a hinge joint with most of its movement in one plane only, flexion and extension. The joint is more stable in dorsiflexion, a point to remember in ankle taping.

Covered by a layer of cartilage, the talus moves anteriorly and posteriorly in the cup-like cavity formed by the distal heads of the tibia and fibula. The talus acts as a movable saddle for the two bones of the lower leg. The talus, in turn, sits forward and on top of the calcaneus. The talus allows forward and downward movement of the ankle. The ankle joint, because of its arrangement of bones attaching ligaments, is structurally very strong. However, because of the stresses of athletics, the ankle is often

injured. In spite of the fact that ankle injuries are relatively common, treatment and rehabilitation are often incomplete.

After the bony structure, the first line of defense against ankle sprains is the joint's strong ligamentous support. Just as with the bony structure, the ligaments of the ankle make the joint more stable laterally. Most of the ligaments involved in supporting the ankle are attached to the rough edges of the malleoli. The ligaments are named for the bones they connect.

It is not necessary for beginning student athletic trainers to learn the names of all the ligaments of the ankle. Those ligaments most commonly injured are the anterior and posterior talofibular (laterally) and the deltoid ligament (medially). The deltoid ligament is actually a group of four ligaments.

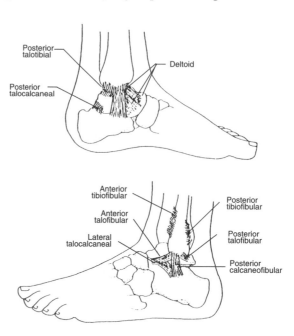

*The ankle joint, because of its arrangement of bones and ligaments, is structurally very strong. However, it is often injured in athletics, requiring complete treatment and rehabilitation before the athlete returns to activity. (source: **Modern Principles of Athletic Training, 6th Ed., Daniel D. Arnheim, 1985**)*

For evaluation purposes, the student athletic trainer should know the location of all the ankle joint ligaments.

Posterior View of Muscles of the lower leg.

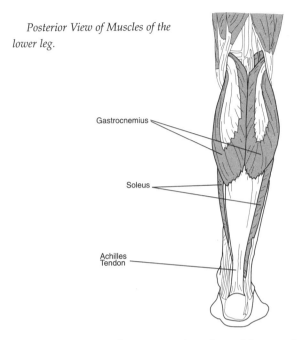

Gastrocnemius

Soleus

Achilles Tendon

The major muscles supporting the ankle are also shown. Two of the muscle tendon groups most important in preventing ankle injuries are the Achilles tendon and the peroneus muscle group.

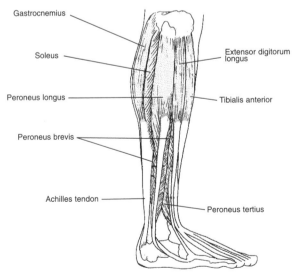

Gastrocnemius

Soleus

Peroneus longus

Peroneus brevis

Achilles tendon

Extensor digitorum longus

Tibialis anterior

Peroneus tertius

Lateral View of muscles of the lower leg. (source: Essentials of Athletic Training, 2nd Ed., Arnheim, 1991.)

A tight Achilles tendon, which is the attachment of the gastrocnemius and soleus muscles (calf muscles) to the calcaneus, is often the cause of recurrent ankle sprains.

The peroneal muscle group runs along the lateral side of the leg and foot, attaching underneath the foot. When the peroneal group contracts, it causes the foot to evert, which helps to prevent a sprain to the lateral ligaments.

This section will deal with the common injuries and conditions of the lower leg. The two bones of the lower leg are the tibia and the smaller and lateral bone, the fibula. The area on the front of the lower leg is called the shin. Often associated with shin pain is the interosseous membrane, which connects the tibia and fibula. There is no large muscle mass on the front of the leg, and the blood supply to it is poor. The most prominent features on the back of the lower leg are the calf muscles (gastrocnemius and soleus) and the Achilles tendon. Often called the heel cord, the Achilles tendon of the calf muscles attaches to the calcaneus, or heel bone.

This area of the body is innervated by a number of different nerves. Those nerves that produce sensory feeling in the region include S1, S2, L4, and L5.

Foot, Ankle, and Lower Leg Anatomy - Bones
- Phalanges
- Metatarsals
- Tarsals
- Tibia
- Fibula

Foot, Ankle, and Lower Leg Anatomy - Ligaments
- Plantar calcaneonavicular ligament
- Posterior talocalcaneal ligament
- Calcaneofibular ligament
- Lateral talocalcaneal ligament
- Anterior talofibular ligament
- Posterior talofibular ligament
- Deltoid ligament

Foot, Ankle, and Lower Leg Anatomy - Muscles
- Extensor and flexor digitorum brevis
- Abductor and adductor hallucis
- Peroneals
- Gastrocnemius
- Soleus
- Tibialis posterior and anterior

Foot, Ankle, and Lower Leg Anatomy - Joints
- Interphalangeal joints
- Metatarsophalangeal joints
- Intermetatarsal joints
- Tarsometatarsal joints
- Intertarsal joints
- Ankle joint

Foot, Ankle and Lower Leg Anatomy - Dermatomes
- S1 - Phalanges and plantar aspect of foot
- S2 - Proximal 1/3 of posterior aspect of lower leg
- L4 - Anteriomedial aspect of lower leg and rear 1/3 of foot
- L5 - Anteriolateral and posterior aspect of lower leg and dorsum of foot

Evaluation Format

The first purpose of an evaluation is to determine, to the best of your ability, if there is a fracture. Initially, a fracture should always be suspected. Signs of a fracture include, but are not limited to, direct or indirect pain, deformity, or a grating sound at the injury site. Some fractures are not accompanied by swelling or pain. If a fracture is suspected, the evaluation stops. The limb is splinted and the athlete is transported to proper medical authorities. Young athletes are especially susceptible to fractures. Often, the ligaments are stronger than the bones. A force that will tear a ligament in a mature athlete will often avulse or pull away a chunk of bone in the younger athlete.

The evaluation process to help determine the type of injury involves four steps: history, observation, palpation, and stress tests.

(H) History: This involves asking questions of the athlete to help determine the mechanism of injury. Answers to these questions will help the physician in a diagnosis.

(O) Observation: Look for bleeding, deformity, swelling, discoloration, and scars. The athletic trainer should compare the injured ankle to the healthy ankle.

(P) Palpation: Any palpation (physical inspection) should take into account the emotional state of the athlete. Palpate the area away from the injury first, working toward the injury site. The entire area around the injury may be sore, but the athletic trainer should try to pinpoint the site of most severe pain. That will be the site where the most damage has been done. From knowledge of the ankle's anatomy, the type and extent of injury can be evaluated. Involve the athlete in the evaluation as much as possible. Asking questions that require specific answers can provide valuable information.

(S) Stress Tests: With all tests, the athletic trainer is looking for pain and instability. Note: It is possible to further damage an injured ankle through manipulation. Years of training are necessary before an athletic trainer would be considered competent to make stress and functional tests. These tests are well beyond the expertise of a student athletic trainer. Functional Tests: To determine if damage has been done to muscles, the athletic trainer uses functional tests, including range of motion. The athlete performs active and resistive exercises through all ranges of motion bilaterally against the athletic trainer's resistance. Pain or weakness could indicate muscle damage.

Refer to Chapter 2 for a full explanation of the H.O.P.S. injury evaluation format.

Assessment Tests

All injured joints should be properly evaluated. The purpose of a thorough evaluation is to enable the allied health professional to properly assess the severity of the injury and make recommendations regarding treatment and possible return to participation. Listed below is a review of evaluation techniques outlined in the *Sports Medicine Evaluation Series: Ankle and Lower Leg* published by Mosby Year Book, and sold by Cramer Products.

Tests for Bony Integrity:
- Heel Tap Test
- Squeeze Test

Tests for Ligamentous Stability:
- Anterior Drawer Test
- Inversion or Lateral Stress Test
- Eversion or Medial Stress Test
- External Rotation Test

Tests for Muscle Function and Flexibility:
- Thompson Test
- Gastrocnemius Tightness Test
- Soleus Tightness Test

Common Injuries
Conditions That Indicate an Athlete Should be Referred for Physician Evaluation
- Gross deformity
- Significant swelling and especially an early hemarthrosis (blood in the joint)

Blisters can be very painful, and even debilitating, if not properly treated. The application of a "donut" pad can help take pressure off a blister

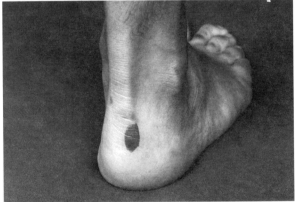

- Loss of motion
- Joint instability
- Significant pain
- Dislocated ankle
- Abnormal sensations such as clicking, popping, grating, or weakness
- Locked ankle or excessively limited motion
- Any doubt regarding the severity or nature of the injury

Blisters: Although blisters can occur on any part of the body where friction occurs, in athletics they are most often found on the feet. As the layers of the skin rub together, friction causes separation. The body responds with fluid formation in this separation. This fluid creates pressure on nerve endings, which is perceived as pain. If the blister is neglected, it may break, creating an open wound.

Once formed, blisters cannot be ignored. Proper treatment of a blister is mandatory in order to insure maximum comfort of the athlete and reduce the possibility of infection. Blisters can be very painful, and even debilitating, if not properly treated.

Arch Sprains: Most people are unaware that there are four arches in the foot. Each contributes to balance, movement, support, and shock absorption. To help understand these arches, place a wet foot down on an absorbent paper towel and observe the footprint.

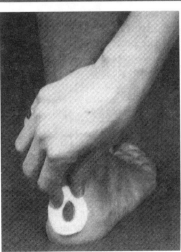 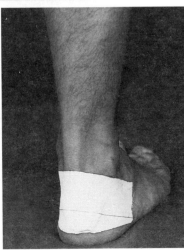 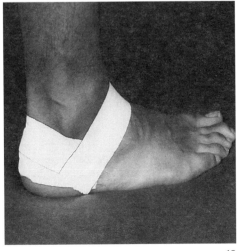

Any of the four arches of the foot (transverse, metatarsal, inner, or outer longitudinal) can suffer supportive ligament sprains. Once the ligaments are stretched, they fail to hold the bones of the foot in position.

When an arch is weakened in this manner, it can not absorb shock as well as it is designed to do. Resulting manifestations the student athletic trainer might see include shin splints, achilles tendon strain, foot fatigue, strained muscles, and even blisters. If the student athletic trainer treats only the symptoms, the arch sprain may worsen.

Causes of arch problems include overuse, overweight, fatigue, training on hard surfaces, and wearing non-supportive, worn shoes. First aid, as with other ligament sprains, includes cold, compression, and elevation. Most arch sprains are to the metatarsal arch (at the distal end of the metatarsals) or inner longitudinal arch.

Plantar Fasciitis: The plantar fascia is a wide, inelastic ligamentous tissue that extends from the anterior portion of the calcaneus to the heads of the metatarsals, supplying support to the arch of the foot.

This tissue can become strained from overuse, unsupportive footwear, a tight Achilles tendon or running on hard surfaces; most often, the cause of plantar fasciitis is chronic irritation. Cross-country and track athletes are prone to overuse injuries in which the plantar fascia is continually strained from running and jumping. Basketball and volleyball athletes are also susceptible to plantar fasciitis from repeated jumping and landing.

An athlete with plantar fasciitis will experience pain and tenderness on the bottom of the foot near the heel. Untreated, this condition causes bone imbalance which can lead to heel spurs, muscle strains, shin splints, and other problems.

Besides treating with cold, the athletic trainer must evaluate and correct the cause of the problem. Taping can help provide support and stability.

Heel Bruise: The heel receives, absorbs, and transfers much of the impact from sports activities, especially running and jumping. Therefore, the ligaments, tendons, and fat pad of the heel are all subject to stress and injury.

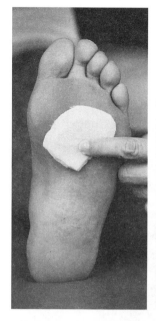
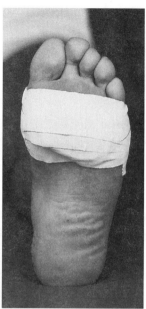
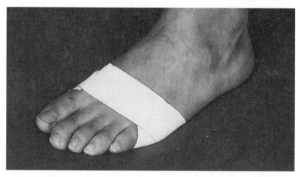

Applying a metatarsal arch pad cushions the sprained arch, helping to relieve pain.

The plantar fascia is a wide band of inelastic tissue that is especially susceptible to injury from overuse or repeated jumping and landing.

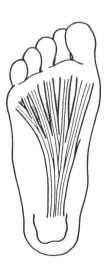

Along with the hip pointer, the heel bruise is among the most disabling contusions in athletics. The protective fat pad must be rested or protected during athletic activity to allow healing to occur. Cold application before activity, and cold and eleva-

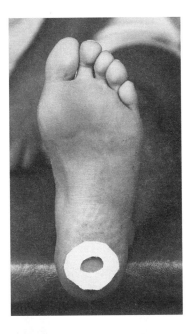

The heel bruise is a very painful injury that requires rest and protection to heal. A donut pad can be applied, as shown here, to help protect the bruised area.

tion afterwards can help reduce swelling and pain.

The athletic trainer can also supply the athlete with heel cups to help absorb the force of the heel's impact with the ground or floor, or a donut pad can be constructed to protect the bruised area. To prevent muscle imbalance and problems from misalignment of the body, both shoes, not just the shoe of the injured foot, should contain equal amounts of padding.

Heel Spur: A heel spur is a bony growth on the calcaneus that causes painful inflammation of the accompanying soft tissue and is aggravated by exercise. The student athletic trainer can locate a heel spur by pressing on the heel. This condition is often caused by "flat feet." As the foot flattens, the plantar fascia is stretched and pulled at the point where it attaches to the calcaneus. Over a period of time, the calcaneus reacts to this irritation by forming a spur of bony material. The team physician may recommend taping the arch or the use of shoe inserts (orthoses) to help reduce the plantar fascia's pull on the calcaneus.

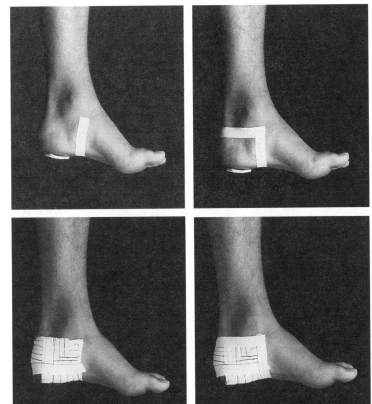

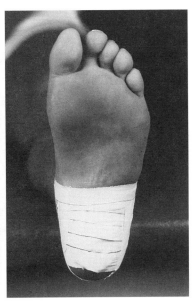

Turf Toe: The great toe is very important in balance, movement, and speed. Occasionally, the ligaments supporting the toe will become sprained, severely limiting the athlete's performance. Turf toe is the name given to such a sprain. Often, the mechanism of the injury will be the foot sliding back on a slippery surface, which forcefully hyperextends the toe.

As with any acute sprain, immediate care of turf toe is application of cold and elevation. The physician may take X-rays to rule out a more severe injury. Most sprains of the great toe are minor. Once normal function returns, the athletic trainer should support the toe to prevent another sprain.

Ankle Sprains: Ankle injuries range from muscle strains and ligament sprains to dislocations and fractures. The most common injury is the sprain; its mechanism of injury is usually a combination of excessive inversion and plantar flexion. The mechanism is similar to an athlete stepping into a hole. More than 80 percent of all ankle sprains are of this type of mechanism. The ligament most often injured is the anterior talofibular. Since most sprains are of the lateral, or inversion type, ankle tapings have been designed to prevent the inversion sprain.

A sample taping method for turf toe.

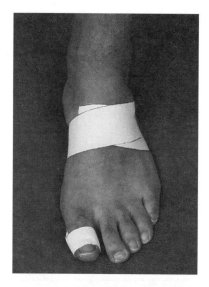
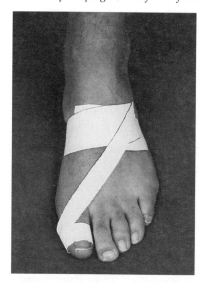
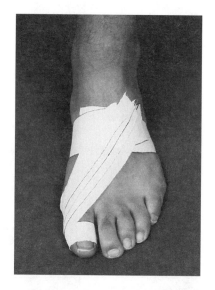
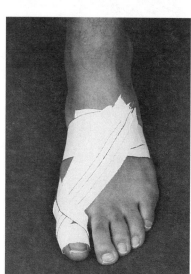
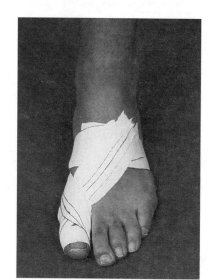
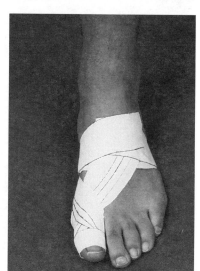

Applying a cold compression wrap to an injured ankle will help speed the healing process.

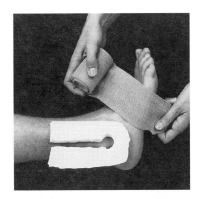

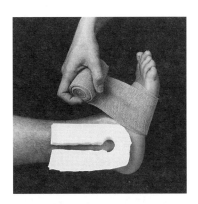

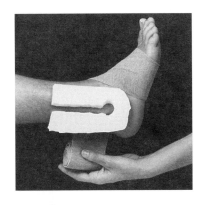

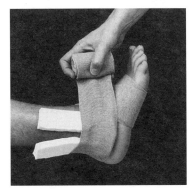

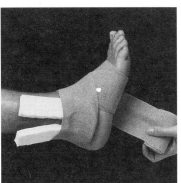

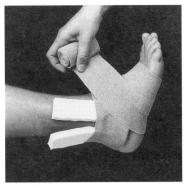

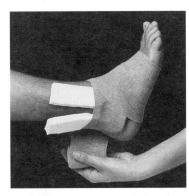

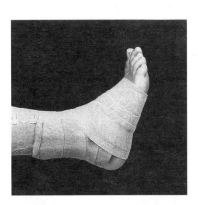

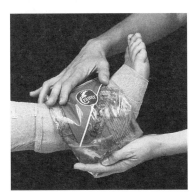

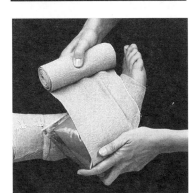

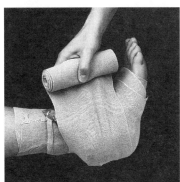

Less common is the eversion sprain. On the medial side of the ankle is the tough, thick deltoid ligament, which helps prevent excessive eversion, or foot-out movement. Whether the sprain is of the inversion or eversion type, it is usually placed into one of three categories: first degree (mild), second degree (moderate), or third degree (severe).

First degree sprain: One or more of the supporting ligaments and surrounding tissues are stretched. There is minor discomfort, point tenderness, and little or no swelling. There is no abnormal movement in the joint to indicate lack of stability.

Second degree sprain: A portion of one or more ligaments is torn. There is pain, swelling, point tenderness, and loss of function for several minutes or longer. There is slight abnormal movement in the joint. The athlete may not be able to walk normally and will favor the injured leg.

Third degree sprain: One or more ligaments have been completely torn, resulting in joint instability. There is either extreme pain or little pain (if nerve damage has occurred), loss of function, point tenderness, and rapid swelling. An accompanying fracture is possible.

Shin Splints: The term shin splints has inaccurately become a catch-all term to describe pain or injury of the anterior portion of the lower leg. However, for the student athletic trainer to assume that any lower leg pain in athletics is a symptom of shin splints would be a mistake. Two other much more serious injuries often have similar symptoms to shin splints. These injuries are stress fractures and anterior compartment syndrome. By determining the mechanism of injury, the athletic trainer can treat the specific injury. The shin splint injury is thought to be an inflammation of the interosseous membrane, strains to the soleus muscle, or other chronic lower leg conditions. Because of the lower leg's poor blood supply, any injury in this region can be slow to heal. Left untreated and uncorrected, the condition can worsen until it is disabling. Some causes of shin splints are suddenly increasing the level of conditioning, muscle weakness or imbalance, lack of proper conditioning, improper or incomplete warmup, poor flexibility or lack of stretching, running on hard surfaces, improper running form or habits, improper or worn running shoes, or poor foot structure.

Stress Fractures: Bones are not inanimate objects. They are living tissue. Just like muscle cells, bone cells respond to exercise, growing stronger to meet new demands. Lack of exercise can lead to deterioration, or deossification of the bone. If the exercise is too severe, or of too long a duration, the change in the bone structure will be negative; a stress fracture can begin to develop. Continued stress will lead to a worsening of the fracture. Because stress fractures often occur in the lower leg, there is a tendency to dismiss pain in this area as mere shin splints. Early X-rays of the shin may not reveal evidence of the stress fracture. A second series of X-rays may be indicated after three weeks to confirm or rule out stress fractures.

Signs of a stress fracture might be increased pain every time the athlete exercises. Point tenderness is also an indicator of an injury more severe than shin splints. Usually, a stress fracture will hurt when the athlete presses with the fingers just above and below the site of most pain. If a stress fracture is suspected, the student athletic trainer should notify the physician. First aid procedures include the application of cold and elevation.

Anterior Compartment Syndrome: Anterior compartment syndrome is another condition that, when suspected by the coach or student athletic trainer, should be referred immediately to the physician.

The lower leg is made up of four compartments: (1) anterior, (2) lateral, (3) superficial posterior and (4) deep posterior. Most compartment syndromes in athletics are to the anterior compartment. As with stress fractures, anterior compartment syndrome can be mistaken for shin splints. In addition, anterior compartment syndrome can be misdiagnosed as a contusion of the shin, muscle cramps, or spasms.

The anterior compartment is tightly filled with the muscles that dorsiflex the foot and ankle. It is almost entirely enclosed with rigid walls of bone or tissue. The danger in misdiagnosis is a worsening of the condition. This could lead to permanent nerve damage, which could result in permanent disability. Direct trauma or excessive exercise can result in hemorrhage and swelling inside the compartment. This swelling will increase the pressure on the peroneal nerve, the veins, and, finally, the arteries inside the compartment. Without arterial circulation, muscle cells will die.

Signs of anterior compartment syndrome include pain even after cold treatment, a firmness of the muscle, numbness of the foot, and warmth. Once suspected, anterior compartment syndrome should be treated as a medical emergency. First aid treatment should be cold in the form of an ice bag or cold pack placed on the injury. Unlike most injuries compression and elevation should not be used, as they could worsen the condition. The pressure of ice massage could also aggravate the injury.

Achilles Tendon Strain: Although the Achilles tendon is the strongest in the body, it is a vulnerable area for athletes; severe damage such as a tear can be career-threatening. The tendon is formed by the union of the gastrocnemius and soleus muscles on the back of the leg; the tendon inserts on the calcaneus. Injuries can be caused by overuse, muscle imbalance inflexibility, or a sudden movement. Depending on the force and the condition of the tendon, the injuries can range from mild strains to complete ruptures.

Strains of this important tendon must be treated more conservatively than most muscle injuries. This is because of the disability the injury produces and the tendency for the strain to develop into a

Rehabilitation

Sending an athlete back to competition before healing is complete leaves the player susceptible to further injury. The best way to determine when healing is complete is by the absence of pain during stressful activity and by the return of full range of motion and strength.

Prior to the beginning of any rehabilitation exercise program, the athletic trainer should consult with a medical doctor to establish an individual program tailored for that individual athlete and the specific injury to be rehabilitated. The following exercises can be used as rehabilitative exercises, or for preventive exercises:

Lower Leg:
- Plantar Flexion
- Dorsi Flexion
- Inversion Tubing
- Eversion Tubing
- Slide Board
- Stationary Bicycle
- Heel Lifts
- Progressive Running Program
- Sport Specific Exercises
- PNF Exercises

Ankle:
- Wedge Board
- BAPS
- Incline Board
- Mini Squats
- Stationary Bicycle
- Progressive Running Program
- Sport Specific Exercises

Foot:
- Towel Gathering
- Sponge Pick Up
- Stationary Bicycle
- Progressive Running Program
- Sport Specific Exercises

Included in any rehabilitation protocol would be the following:
- Range-of-Motion Exercises
- Resistance Exercises
- Sport Specific Exercises

complete tear. The Achilles tendon is sometimes strained when the ankle is sprained, and may take longer to heal than the injured ligaments. A strong, stable, and flexible Achilles tendon can prevent many ankle sprains. Strains are treated with cold, compression, and elevation. Follow-up treatments can include cold, heat, or contrast baths.

Muscle Cramps: In athletics, athletic trainers often see an athlete make a rapid recovery from what appears to be a painful, disabling knee or ankle injury. In those cases, the injury may simply be a cramp in the calf muscles. (Other muscles can also cramp involuntarily, but the calf muscles are especially susceptible.) A cramp is a sudden, violent contraction of a muscle. While the cause is unknown, several factors seem to contribute to their incidence:
- Overwork in early season
- Fatigue
- Loss of fluid from perspiration
- Poor foot structure which causes tension and strain on muscles and tendons
- Lack of proper nutrients in the diet
- Incomplete rehabilitation of a previous injury
- Improperly fitted equipment or shoes that retard circulation, preventing complete relaxation of the muscles
- Imbalance in the lumbar area of the low back, aggravated by improper strain
- Poor flexibility
- Fractures

Preventive/Supportive Techniques

Taping is a time-honored and time-consuming tradition. It is also a very expensive practice. Whether to tape healthy body parts is a decision the athletic trainer will have to make.

All injured joints should be taped initially. The purpose of taping is to keep the joint from moving so the ligaments would not be stretched further.

Foot:
- Great Toe Taping
- Heel Taping
- Metatarsal Arch Pad with Taping
- Inner Longitudinal Arch Taping
- Toe Splint Taping
- Plantar Fasciitis Taping

Ankle:
- Ankle Taping
- Open Basket Weave Taping
- Cloth Ankle Wrap

Lower Leg:
- Shin Splint Taping
- Achilles Tendon Taping

NATA Competency Terms

Listed below is a list of musculoskeletal conditions/disorders that affect the ankle, foot and /or lower leg. A valuable learning experience would be to define and review these conditions in a medical dictionary and/or sports medicine textbook.

- Achilles Tendon Rupture

- Ankle Sprain

- Ankle Sprain/Fracture

- Exotoses

- Fracture (tibia, fibula, tarsals, metatarsals, etc.)

- Great Toe Sprain (Turf Toe)

- Ingrown Toenail

- Plantar Faciitis

- Shin Splints

- Stress Fractures (tibia, fibula, metatarsals)

- Tendinitis/Tenosynovitis

Chapter 6 - Review Questions

Completion:

1. The _____ is mounted almost directly on top of the talus and extends overs its medial side.

2. The _____ _____ is actually a group of four ligaments.

3. If a fracture is suspected, the evaluation _____.

4. The athletic trainer should compare the injured ankle to the _____ _____.

5. _____ _____ refers to a sprain of the ligaments that support the great toe.

6. Prior to the beginning of any rehabilitation programs, the athletic trainer should _____.

7. _____ _____ usually refers to a great toe sprain.

8. The strongest tendon in this body part is the _____ _____.

9. The four arches of the foot are the _____, _____, _____ _____, and the _____ _____.

10. Factors that contribute to muscle cramps are _____, _____, _____, and _____.

11. Absence of _____ and full _____ __ _____ during stressful activity are signs of healing of an injury.

12. Taping keeps _____ from moving and _____ from stretching.

13. Two indicators of stress fractures are _____ and _____.

14. Of the two major bones of the lower leg, the _____ is larger than the _____.

15. The two most prominent features on the back of the leg are the calf muscles (the _____ and the _____) and the _____ tendon, also known as the heel cord.

16. The term, shin splints, is often used to describe pain of the _____ portion of the lower leg.

17. Because shin splints is an inflammation, _____ is the most effective treatment after exercise.

18. The Thompson test is used to determine if the _____ _____ is ruptured.

19. The large, bony protrusions on each side of the ankle are known as the _____.

20. The four bones that form the ankle joint are the _____, _____, _____, and _____.

21. With inversion ankle sprains, the ligament most often injured is the _____ _____ ligament, on the _____ side of the ankle.

22. When evaluating an eversion ankle sprain, a fracture of the _____ should be suspected.

23. If an athlete with an ankle injury can't walk without a limp, _____ should be used.

Short Answer:

1. Define the acronym HOPS.
-
-
-
-

2. Define the three types of sprains.
-
-
-

3. Name two tests for bony integrity:
-
-

4. Name two tests for ligamentous stability:
-
-

5. Name the two most commonly injured arches of the foot:
-
-

6. Name two foot taping techniques:
-
-

7. Name two types of ankle taping techniques:
-
-

8. Name two NATA competency terms:
-
-

9. List the four arches of the foot:

•

•

•

•

10. Identify a test for bony integrity.

11. Identify a muscle function test.

12. Identify some of the exercises used to rehabilitate the ankle.

13. Define an Achilles tendon rupture.

14. Define a great toe sprain.

15. What is the best way to determine when healing is complete?

16. What is the most common ankle injury in athletics? What is its mechanism of injury?

17. Why are eversion ankle sprains less likely to occur than inversion sprains?

18. What are the symptoms of anterior compartment syndrome?

19. What common chronic conditions may be caused by excessive running?

20. How are stress fractures evaluated and managed?

NOTES

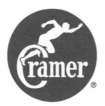

Chapter 7

The Knee, Quadriceps and Hamstrings

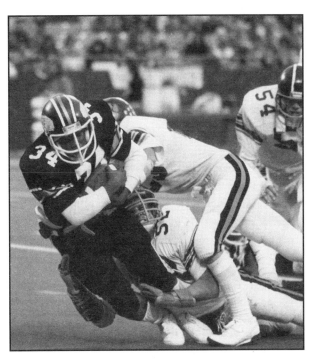

Educational Objectives

The learner should, at the completion of the chapter, be able to perform the following:

- Understand the anatomy of the knee, quadriceps, and hamstrings.
- Recognize the steps in an evaluation format.
- Identify the assessment tests for injuries to this part of the lower extremity.
- Recognize the common injuries to this part of the lower extremity.
- Understand the principles of rehabilitation to this part of the body.
- Understand the components of taping and wrapping to this part of the body.
- Recognize the NATA competencies for this section of the body.

The knee is a complicated joint and injuries can be complex. After first aid for most knee injuries physician referral is recommended.

Fortunately, it has been found that many of the more serious knee injuries in sports can be prevented. The key is that the athlete work to strengthen the quadriceps and hamstring muscle groups. For those injuries that do occur, knees that are protected by strong muscles often suffer less severe problems. Rehabilitation time is also reduced if the knee musculature is strong to begin with.

Anatomy

The knee is the largest joint in the body. Despite its size, though, it is structurally very weak. The joint's primary weakness is due to its relatively unstable bony structure. To illustrate this instability, consider the femur, or thigh bone. The femur is the longest and strongest bone in the body. However, it

sits precariously on top of the smaller tibia, which is the main weight-bearing bone of the lower leg. These two bones slide back and forth on each other, even in non-stressful, non-athletic activities. Subtracting further from the joint's stability is the small amount of normal rotation by the femur on the tibia.

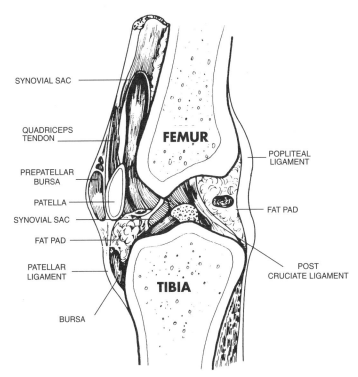

Although the knee is the largest joint in the body, it is very weak because of its relatively unstable bone structure.

Not everything in this joint's structure is detrimental to stability, though. The distal end of the femur has two slightly convex surfaces, called condyles. These condyles articulate with the slightly concave surfaces of the tibia. However, once the knee starts to bend, whether the action is walking, running, or climbing stairs, what little contribution to stability these convex and concave surfaces have is greatly diminished.

The femur and tibia are only two of the four bones of the knee joint. The next largest bone is the fibula, the non-weight-bearing bone of the lower leg. The fibula articulates at the knee only with the tibia, and serves as the attachment for the lateral collateral ligament.

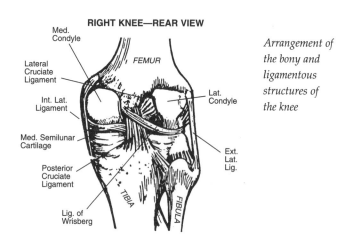

RIGHT KNEE—REAR VIEW

Med. Condyle
Lateral Cruciate Ligament
FEMUR
Int. Lat. Ligament
Lat. Condyle
Med. Semilunar Cartilage
Posterior Cruciate Ligament
Ext. Lat. Lig.
TIBIA
FIBULA
Lig. of Wrisberg

Arrangement of the bony and ligamentous structures of the knee

The fourth bone of the knee joint is called the patella, or knee cap. The patella, encased in the powerful patellar tendon, moves up and down in front of the knee in the space between the two condyles of the femur.

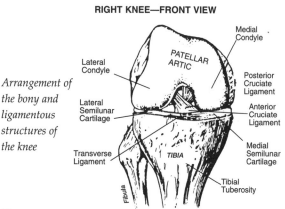

RIGHT KNEE—FRONT VIEW

Arrangement of the bony and ligamentous structures of the knee

Lateral Condyle
PATELLAR ARTIC
Medial Condyle
Posterior Cruciate Ligament
Lateral Semilunar Cartilage
Anterior Cruciate Ligament
Transverse Ligament
Medial Semilunar Cartilage
TIBIA
Fibula
Tibial Tuberosity

The instability of the knee's bony structure is partially compensated for by strong ligaments and potentially even stronger muscle support. Four important ligaments help stabilize the knee: the medial collateral ligament, the lateral collateral ligament, and the anterior and posterior cruciate ligaments.

On the medial side of the knee, the broad, flat medial collateral ligament (MCL) helps secure the femur to the tibia. It also connects to the cartilage of the knee, the medial meniscus. Located on the other side of the knee, the lateral collateral ligament (LCL) is not quite as strong as the medial ligament. The LCL is cord-like, rather than a broad band. Unlike the MCL, the LCL does not attach to the lateral meniscus.

The two cruciate ligaments form an "x" in the center the joint (cruciate comes from the Latin word meaning cross). These ligaments restrict anterior and posterior movement of the femur on the tibia.

More than any other joint, the knee is dependent on good muscle support. In fact, there are 13 muscles that support the knee. Most of the support comes from the large muscle groups of the thigh (both front and back) as well as the gastrocnemius muscle of the lower leg. These supporting muscle groups are the quadriceps (on the front of the thigh) and the hamstrings (on the back of the thigh).

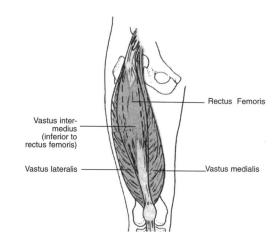

Rectus Femoris
Vastus intermedius (inferior to rectus femoris)
Vastus lateralis
Vastus medialis

*Quadricep muscle group (source: **Essentials of Athletic Training, 3rd Ed., Daniel D. Arnheim, 1995**)*

The quadriceps muscles, which extend (straighten) the lower leg, converge to form the patellar tendon. As mentioned earlier, this tendon encases the patella. The quadriceps insert on the front of the tibia on the tibial tubercle.

The hamstring muscle group flexes (bends) the leg and also helps control the rotary movements of the tibia. Called a natural knee brace by many athletic trainers, the hamstrings originate on the pelvis and femur and divide to attach below the knee on the tibia and fibula. While the quadriceps and hamstrings are of greatest concern to the athletic trainer and coach, other muscles also provide support and control movement of the knee. These muscles include the adductors, abductors, and the gastrocnemius.

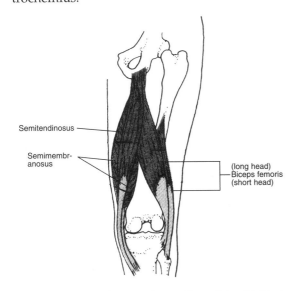

*Hamstring muscle group (source: **Essentials of Athletic Training, 3rd Ed., Daniel D. Arnheim, 1995**)*

The knee joint contains two tough, fibrous cartilages, known as menisci. They are called the lateral meniscus and medial meniscus. These menisci rest on top of the tibia in its two shallow concave indentations. The menisci form a cushioned base for the medial and lateral condyles of the femur. Other functions of the menisci include shock-absorption, adding to joint stability and helping to smooth the gliding and rotating movements of the femur and tibia.

Other structures in the knee of special concern in athletics are the bursae and the synovial membrane. The bursae (there are about 13 in the area of the knee) are closed, fluid-filled sacs. These sacs serve as cushions against friction over a prominent bone, or where a tendon moves over a bone. The synovial membrane is a large, closed sac that lines the inside of the knee joint, helping to lubricate the tendons, ligaments, and bones.

Knee Anatomy - Bones
- Femur
- Tibia
- Fibula
- Patella

Knee Anatomy - Ligaments
- Anterior Cruciate Ligament
- Posterior Cruciate Ligament
- Medial Collateral Ligament
- Lateral Collateral Ligament
- Ligament of Wrisberg
- Transverse Ligament

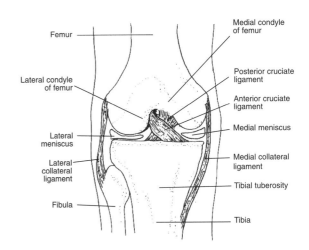

*The anterior view of the bony and ligamentous arrangement of the knee. (source: **Essentials of Athletic Training, 3rd Ed., Daniel D. Arnheim, 1995**)*

Knee Anatomy - Muscles

- Vastus Medialis
- Vastus Lateralis
- Vastus Intermedius
- Rectus Femoris
- Gracilis
- Sartorius
- Semitendinosus
- Semimembranosus
- Popliteus
- Gastrocnemius

Knee Anatomy - Joints

- Hinge joint
- Diarthroses

Dermatomes

- L2 - Quadriceps and lateral hamstring
- L3 - Knee and medial hamstring
- S2 - Middle hamstring

Evaluation Format

The first purpose of an evaluation is to determine, to the best of your ability, if there is a fracture. Initially, a fracture should always be suspected. Signs of a fracture include, but are not limited to, direct or indirect pain, deformity, or a grating sound at the injury site. Some fractures are not accompanied by swelling or pain. If a fracture is suspected, the evaluation stops. The limb is splinted and the athlete is transported to proper medical authorities. Young athletes are especially susceptible to fractures. Often, the ligaments are stronger than the bones. A force that will tear a ligament in a mature athlete will often avulse or pull away a chunk of bone in the younger athlete.

The evaluation process to help determine the type of injury involves four steps: history, observation, palpation, and stress tests.

(H) History: This involves asking questions of the athlete to help determine the mechanism of injury. Answers to these questions will help the physician in a diagnosis.

(O) Observation: Look for bleeding, deformity, swelling, discoloration and scars. The athletic trainer should compare the injured area to the uninjured area.

(P) Palpation: Any palpation (physical inspection) should take into account the emotional state of the athlete. Palpate the area away from the injury first, working towards the injury site. The entire area around the injury may be sore, but the athletic trainer should try to pinpoint the site of most severe pain. That will be the site where the most damage has been done. From knowledge of the knee's anatomy, the type and extent of injury can be evaluated. Involve the athlete in the evaluation as much as possible. Asking questions that require specific answers can provide valuable information.

(S) Stress Tests: With all tests, the athletic trainer is looking for pain and instability. Note: It is possible to further damage an injured knee through manipulation. Years of training are necessary before an athletic trainer would be considered competent to make stress tests and functional tests. These tests are well beyond the expertise of a student athletic trainer. Functional Tests: To determine if damage has been done to muscles, the athletic trainer uses functional tests, including range of motion. The athlete performs active and resistive exercises through all ranges of motion bilaterally against the athletic trainer's resistance. Pain or weakness could indicate muscle damage.

Refer to Chapter 2 for a full explanation of the H.O.P.S. injury evaluation format.

Assessment Tests

All injured joints should be properly evaluated. The purpose of a thorough evaluation is to enable the allied health professional to properly assess the severity of the injury and make recommendations regarding treatment and possible return to participation. Listed below is a review of evaluation techniques outlined in the *Sports Medicine Evaluation Series: The Knee* published by Mosby Year Book, and distributed by Cramer Products.

Tests for knee ligament stability:
- Abduction or valgus stress test
- Adduction or varus stress test
- Anterior drawer test
- Posterior drawer test
- Lachman's test
- Pivot shift test

Tests for knee joint effusion:
- Knee joint test for minor effusion
- Ballotable patella

Tests for patellar stability:
- Apprehension test
- Patella compression test

Tests for meniscal stability:
- McMurray test
- Apley's compression test

Common Injuries
Conditions That Indicate an Athlete Should be Referred for Physician Evaluation
- Gross deformity
- Significant swelling and especially an early hemarthrosis
- Loss of motion
- Joint instability
- Significant pain
- Dislocated patella
- Abnormal sensations such as clicking, popping, grating, or weakness
- Locked knee or excessively limited motion
- Any doubt regarding the severity or nature of the injury

Because the knee does not operate only as a hinge joint — the femur also rotates and slides on the tibia — there are several ways the joint can become injured. And when an injury occurs, chances of it requiring surgery are much greater than with any other joint in the body. Coaches and student athletic trainers should not try to determine whether a knee injury is minor or more severe. Without medical training, an evaluation is not possible. It is possible for a knee to be severely injured and exhibit little swelling or pain; therefore, knee injuries call for immediate referral to a physician.

In athletics, the most common knee injuries are contusions, ligament sprains and torsion injuries.

Contusion injuries are caused by a direct blow or by falling on the knee. Besides muscular contusions, direct blows or falls can also damage the bursae that protect the bones and other structures of the knee. Athletes are likely to suffer knee contusions in basketball, volleyball, wrestling, and football.

Ligament sprains can be caused by blows from any direction and are compounded when the athlete's foot is planted. Most knee sprains occur in football when a player is struck on the lateral side of the leg. In this type of injury, the medial ligament is usually stretched and/or torn.

Torsion injuries occur when the feet are fixed and the body is twisted. This type of injury happens mostly in football. The longer the cleat on the shoe, the greater the risk of torsion injury. A blow severe enough to cause ligament damage will often result in some excessive torsion. Torsion injuries sometimes damage the ligaments, but most often involve the menisci.

Other, usually less severe, knee injuries can be caused by muscular weakness or imbalance, overuse, or repetition; poor running mechanics; or improperly fitted shoes. In addition, some athletes are susceptible to certain knee conditions that are related to the growth process.

Patellar Tendinitis: The patellar tendon emanates from the quadriceps muscles. One of the primary movements of the quadriceps is lower leg extension. This movement is part of the jumping process and the forces generated can be great. The stress that jumping and kicking place on the patellar tendon can cause inflammation just above or below the patella.

Pain is usually reported by the athlete after exercising; some swelling may be present. Use cold to reduce pain and inflammation. The physician may also prescribe rest. As with many knee problems, strong and flexible hamstrings and quadriceps muscles often can prevent or alleviate patellar tendinitis.

Chondromalacia Patellae: Chondromalacia patellae is a painful degenerative condition that results in the irritation and softening of the cartilage of the back of the patella. Running, jumping, kneeling, and climbing stairs can elicit the pain. One cause of this condition is muscular weakness or imbalance. This can cause the patella to track off center as it moves in the femoral groove.

Other causes of chondromalacia patellae are related to the individual athlete's body structure. Whether the cause is muscular or structural, strengthening the quadriceps through straight leg raises and limited range of motion resistance exercises can often correct the problem. Other treatments include cold application before and after activity, isometric strengthening exercises, and use of knee pads.

The Female Athlete's Knee: Because of the structural difference in pelvic girdle width between males and females, patellar problems may be more prevalent for women than men. The female's wider pelvis creates a sharper angle where the femur attaches to the pelvis. This sharper angle changes the line of pull of the quadriceps muscles and may cause the patella to be pulled in a lateral direction upon muscle contraction. This change in mechanics can cause chronic conditions such as chondromalacia patellae, patellar dislocation, or subluxation.

If a female athlete is suffering from one of these chronic knee injuries, strengthening the medial portion of the quadriceps (the vastus medialis) will usually prevent any lateral sliding of the patella. The vastus medialis muscle group can be strengthened by performing complete range of motion resistance exercises. If chronic knee pain persists, refer the athlete to the team physician. The team physician may also recommend ice massage before and after activity, or rest and modification of activity.

Osgood-Schlatter's: The Osgood-Schlatter's condition is common to adolescent males and is characterized by swelling below one or both knees. It involves the growth center of the tibial tubercle to which the patellar tendon attaches. Depending on its severity, the Osgood-Schlatter condition can lead to permanent knee damage.

Osgood-Schlatter condition was first described early in this century as a partial separation of the tibial tubercle from the tendon. Later, it was described as an inflammation of the tibial tubercle, rather than a bone separation. Whatever the cause, this inflammation is aggravated by activity and relieved by rest. Tenderness tends to be most marked at the patellar tendon's insertion point. The athlete will complain of severe pain on jumping, running, or kneeling, and after athletic activity.

In cases of long duration, the front of the knee appears enlarged and a bony prominence can be felt. Although Osgood-Schlatter symptoms disappear after adolescence, this bony prominence remains. The athlete's physician may recommend treatment ranging from restriction or modification of sports activity to immobilization in a cast.

Osgood-Schlatter Condition

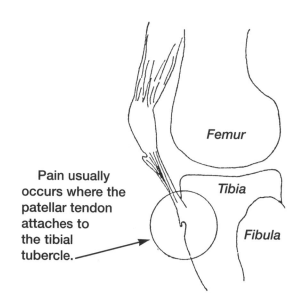

Pain usually occurs where the patellar tendon attaches to the tibial tubercle.

Femur

Tibia

Fibula

Rehabilitation

Regardless of the mechanism of injury, the student athletic trainer's response to knee injuries is basic first aid: compression, cold, and elevation, followed by referral to a physician. Start applying the elastic wrap below the knee, wrapping toward the heart. Then, cold should be applied all around the joint. With support below the knee, the athlete's entire leg should be elevated. The physician's guidelines may call for the use of crutches by the athlete until the examination is made. Delaying referral to a physician for examination and treatment may reduce the chance of the athlete making a complete recovery. As stated above, the best way to prevent knee injuries is through muscle development. It is recommended that all athletes have the strength of their quadriceps and hamstring muscle groups checked. The larger and older the athlete, the stronger these muscle groups need to be.

Typically, the quadriceps of young athletes are much stronger than the hamstrings. To help prevent knee injuries, it is recommended that the hamstrings be at least half as strong as the quadriceps. Within the last few years, the emphasis placed on hamstring strength has played a large role in preventing knee injuries.

Muscle balance, as well as strength, is necessary to prevent injury. During strength training, the athlete should work to have the strength of the corresponding muscle group of the left leg equal to that of the right leg. The only way to build this strength is through resistance exercises or weight training. As with all muscles, strength is lost if the muscle is not exercised regularly. It is therefore important that athletes perform strengthening exercises in-season as well as during the off-season. The physician should recommend a specific knee rehabilitation program, depending on the injury. The student athletic trainer can help supervise the athlete's progress toward recovery.

Before returning to competition, the following rehabilitation guidelines must be met:
- No pain during running, jumping, or cutting
- Full range of motion
- Muscular strength must be equal to that of the uninjured leg
- Strength increase in proportion to the athlete's size and sport

Prior to the beginning of any rehabilitation exercise program, the athletic trainer should consult with a medical doctor to establish an individual program tailored for that individual athlete and the specific injury to be rehabilitated. The following exercises can be used as rehabilitation exercises or for preventive exercises:

Knee:
- Straight Leg Raises
- Terminal Knee Extensions
- Quadriceps Tightening
- Leg Curls
- Leg Extensions
- Stationary Bicycle
- Progressive Running Program
- Sport Specific Exercises

Quadriceps:
- Leg Extensions
- Straight Leg Raises
- Stationary Bicycle
- Progressive Running Program
- Sport Specific Exercises

Hamstrings:
- Leg Curls
- Stationary Bicycle
- Progressive Running Program
- Sport Specific Exercises

Included in any rehabilitation protocol would be the following:
- Range-of-Motion Exercises
- Resistance Exercises
- Sport Specific Exercises

Preventive/Supportive Techniques

Taping is a time-honored and time-consuming tradition. It is also a very expensive practice. Whether to tape healthy body parts is a decision the athletic trainer will have to make.

All injured joints should be taped initially. The purpose of taping is to keep the joint from moving so the ligaments won't be stretched further. Listed below is a review of techniques that are outlined in *The Comprehensive Manual of Taping and Wrapping Techniques* published by Cramer Products.

Knee:
- Collateral Knee Taping
- Hyperextended Knee Taping
- Continuous Figure of Eight Wrap
- Anterior Cruciate Taping
- Patella Tendon Taping

Quadriceps and Hamstrings:
- Elastic Wrap for Quadriceps
- Elastic Wrap for Hamstrings

NATA Competency Terms

Listed below is a list of musculoskeletal conditions/disorders that affect the knee, quadriceps, and/or hamstrings. A valuable learning experience would be to define and review these conditions in a medical dictionary and/or sports medicine textbook.

- Bursitis (suprapatella, infrapatella, etc.)

- Chondromalacia (patella)

- Dislocation (patella, knee)

- Fracture (patella, tibia, fibula)

- Meniscal Tear

- Osgood-Schlatters Disease

- Sprain

- Tendinitis (patella, popliteus, etc.)

Chapter 7 - Review Questions

Completion:

1. After first aid for most knee injuries, referral to a _____ is recommended.

2. The key to preventing many knee injuries involves _____ the _____ and _____ muscle groups.

3. The knee is the largest joint in the body; structurally it is very _____.

4. The main weight bearing bone of the lower leg is the _____.

5. The non-weight bearing bone of the lower leg is the _____.

6. The patella is encased in the powerful patellar _____.

7. The _____ ligaments prevent side-to-side movement of the knee, while the _____ ligaments restrict front-to-back movements.

8. Muscle _____, as well as strength, is necessary to prevent knee injury.

9. The strongest muscle group in the body is the _____ group. The four muscles that compose this group are the _____, _____, _____, and the _____.

10. Swelling caused by synovial fluid or blood in the joint is called _____?

11. _____ knee sprains result from a varus stress to the articular capsule and/or _____ collateral ligament.

12. _____-_____ disease is an apophysitis related to the epiphyseal growth center at the tibial tubercle.

13. Sudden or repetitive forceful extension of the knee may begin an inflammatory process on the patellar tendon, often causing a condition called _____ _____.

14. The largest sesamoid bone in the body is the _____.

Short Answer:

1. What is the largest joint in the body?

2. The two cruciate ligaments in the center of the knee form what shape?

3. What is the purpose of an evaluation?

4. What is the importance of the observation step?

5. What is the adduction stress test?

6. What angle should the knee be flexed in performing the Drawer Test?

7. In athletics, what is the most common knee injury?

8. How is a torsion injury caused?

9. What are the factors under basic first aid for a knee injury?

10. Before beginning a rehabilitation program, what should the athletic trainer do?

11. What is the purpose of taping?

12. What are the preventive/supportive techniques for the quadriceps and hamstrings?

13. Which muscle group is sometimes referred to as the "natural knee brace"?

14. What are the functions of the menisci?

15. What should a student athletic trainer do for most acute knee injuries?

16. Explain why most knee ligament injuries in football are to the medial side.

17. Describe the Osgood-Schlatter condition. Why is it common to adolescents?

18. Are the hamstrings more likely to be contused or strained? Why?

19. Are the quadriceps more likely to be contused or strained? Why?

20. Why should a player who has suffered from a thigh contusion be removed from the game?

21. Describe the proper treatment of a thigh contusion.

22. During flexion and extension what changes occur to the capsular ligaments and cruciate ligaments?

23. In evaluating a knee injury, what questions might the athletic trainer ask the athlete to obtain about the history of the injury and the mechanism that injured it?

24. What are the common tests to determine if a torn meniscus is present? How are they performed?

25. What criteria would be used to determine when the athlete is ready to return to sports participation?

26. Name the four bones of the knee joint.
-
-
-
-

27. Name the four most important ligaments of the knee.
-
-
-
-

28. Name the three hamstring muscles.
-
-
-

29. List four common causes of hamstrings strains.
-
-
-
-

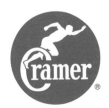

NOTES

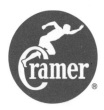

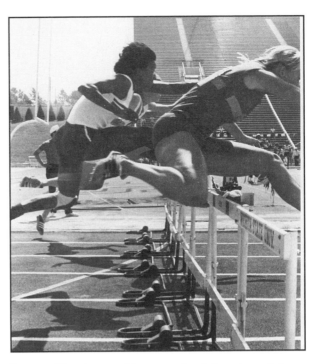

Chapter 8
The Hip and Pelvis

Educational Objectives

The learner should, at the completion of the chapter, be able to perform the following:

- Understand the anatomy of the hip and pelvis.
- Recognize the components of an injury evaluation format.
- Identify the common injuries associated with this body region.
- Identify the protocol for a rehabilitation program to this part of the body.
- Understand the principles of taping and wrapping this body area.
- Recognize the NATA competencies for the hip and pelvis.

Anatomy

One reason there are few sports injuries involving the hip is the strength of the area. Its strong arrangement of bones, muscles, and ligaments makes the hip the strongest joint in the body. The hip joint is a classic ball and socket joint. It is formed by the spherical head of the femur fitting into the deep socket of the hip. There are three parts of the hip: the ilium, the ischium and the pubis. The hip and two sets of fused vertebrae make up the pelvis. These vertebrae are called the sacrum and coccyx. You will remember that some of the muscles that move the leg attach to the pelvis. Also attached to the pelvis are the groin muscles and various muscles involved in supporting and moving the trunk.

Hip - Bones

The bones of the hip and pelvic region provide the structure to transfer weight between the torso and the lower extremities. Those bones include the following:

Femur

Pelvis: Composed of three parts:
    Ilium
    Ischium
    Pubis

Lower Vertebrae: Composed of fused vertebrae divided into two parts:
    Sacrum
    Coccyx

Thigh and Hip - Muscles and Function

There are a number of important muscle groups that are located at the hip and pelvic region. The principal muscles are listed. The largest group of these muscles include the gluteal muscles. These include the gluteus medius, gluteus minimus, and the gluteus maximus. They help with hip extension, internal rotation, and abduction. Another muscle that assists in movement of the hip is the iliopsoas, which has as its primary function hip flexion. Hip flexion is also accomplished by assistance of the tensor fascia latea, sartorius, and pectineus. Hip adduction is performed by the group of muscles known as the adductors. The hip adductor group is composed of adductor longus, adductor brevis, and adductor magnus.

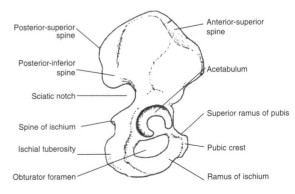

*Pelvis (Source: **Principles of Athletic Training, 8th Ed.,** Arnheim, 1993.)*

The muscle groups that compose the bulk of the thigh (quadriceps and hamstrings) also assist in the movement of the hip. Those movements are hip flexion and hip extension, respectively.

Hip - Ligaments

The principle ligaments of the region include:
• Ligamentum teres
• Transverse acetabular ligament
• Iliofemoral ligament
• Pubofemoral ligament

These are some of the strongest ligaments in the human body. Because of the structure of the bones and muscles, the hip is one of the strongest and least injured areas of the body.

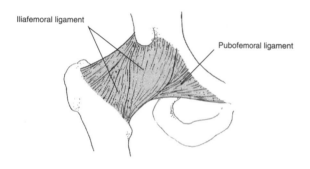

*Ligaments of the hip (source: **Essentials of Athletic Training**, 3rd Ed., Daniel D. Arnheim, 1995.)*

Hip and Thigh - Muscles

• Gluteus medius
• Gluteus minimus
• Gluteus maximus
• Iliopsoas
• Tensor fascia latea
• Sartorius
• Pectineus
• Adductor longus
• Adductor brevis
• Adductor magnus

Hip - Joint

• Ball and Socket joint

Dermatomes

Those nerves that supply sensation to the hip and pelvic region of the body include the following:
• L1 - Upper anterior thigh
• L2 - Lateral and anterior mid thigh
• L3 - Medial thigh
• S2 - Posterior thigh

Evaluation Format

The first purpose of an evaluation is to determine, to the best of your ability, if there is a fracture. Initially, a fracture should always be suspected. Signs of a fracture include, but are not limited to, direct or indirect pain, deformity, or a grating sound at the injury site. Some fractures are not accompanied by swelling or pain. If a fracture is suspected, the evaluation stops. The limb is splinted and the athlete is transported to proper medical authorities. Young athletes are especially susceptible to fractures. Often, the ligaments are stronger than the bones. A force that will tear a ligament in a mature athlete will often avulse or pull away a chunk of bone in the younger athlete.

The evaluation process to help determine the type of injury involves four steps: history, observation, palpation, and stress tests.

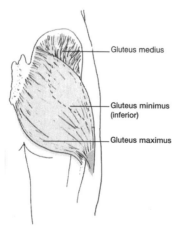

*Gluteal Muscles (source: **Essentials of Athletic Training**, 3rd Ed., Daniel D. Arnheim, 1995.)*

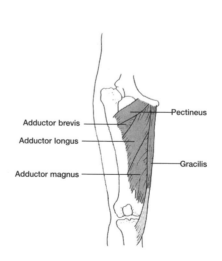

*Hip Adductors (source: **Essentials of Athletic Training**, 3rd Ed., Daniel D. Arnheim, 1995.)*

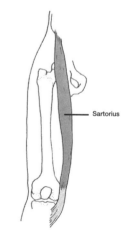

*Satoreous (source: **Essentials of Athletic Training**, 3rd Ed., Daniel D. Arnheim, 1995.)*

(H) History: This involves asking questions of the athlete to help determine the mechanism of injury. Answers to these questions will help the physician in a diagnosis.

(O) Observation: Look for bleeding, deformity, swelling, discoloration, and scars. The athletic trainer should compare the injured hip to the non-injured hip.

(P) Palpation: Any palpation (physical inspection) should take into account the emotional state of the athlete. Palpate the area away from the injury first, working toward the injury site. The entire area around the injury may be sore, but the athletic trainer should try to pinpoint the site of most severe pain. That will be the site where the most damage has been done. From knowledge of the hip's anatomy, the type and extent of injury can be evaluated. Involve the athlete in the evaluation as much as possible. Asking questions that require specific answers can provide valuable information.

(S) Stress Tests: With all tests, the athletic trainer is looking for pain and instability. Note: It is possible to further damage an injured hip joint through manipulation. Years of training are necessary before an athletic trainer would be considered competent to make stress tests and functional tests. These tests are well beyond the expertise of a student athletic trainer. Functional Tests: To determine if damage has been done to muscles, the athletic trainer uses functional tests, including range of motion. The athlete performs active and resistive exercises through all ranges of motion bilaterally against the athletic trainer's resistance. Pain or weakness could indicate muscle damage.

Refer to Chapter 2 for a full explanation of the H.O.P.S. injury evaluation format.

Assessment Test

All injured joints should be properly evaluated. The purpose of a thorough evaluation is to enable the allied health professional to properly assess the severity of the injury and make recommendations regarding treatment and possible return to participation. Listed below is a review of evaluation techniques for the hip and pelvis.

Tests for Bony Integrity:
- Compression Test - Anterior/Posterior force
- Compression Test - Lateral /Medial force

Tests for Muscle Function:
- Knee Extension
- Hip Flexion
- Hip Extension
- Hip Adduction
- Hip Abduction

Tests for Flexibility:
- Hip Flexor Stretch
- Quadricep Stretch
- Hamstring Stretch
- Low Back Flexion Stretches
- Low Back Extension Stretches

Common Injuries
Conditions That Indicate an Athlete Should be Referred for Physician Evaluation
- Gross deformity or swelling
- Significant loss of motion
- Severe disability
- Noticeable and palpable deficit in the muscle or tendon
- Tenderness palpated at the bony attachments
- Continued or severe pain in the hip
- Thigh or hip injury that does not respond to treatment within two to three weeks
- Any doubt regarding the severity or nature of the injury

Injury to the coccyx: The four fused vertebrae on the lower end of the spine are called the coccyx, or tail bone. Often, this area is bruised from falling on a hard surface. Most injuries to the coccyx will be contusions, although severe trauma could cause a dislocation or fracture. Contusions, of course, are treated with cold (i.e., ice packs).

Hip Strains: This injury occurs because of violent twisting motions of the torso and accompanied by the feet being fixed. The evaluation is best determined with the athlete being unable to circumduct the thigh.

Trochanteric Bursitis: This common hip problem is also called bursitis. It usually occurs in the region of the gluteus medius or the iliotibial band. Running technique should be examined as well as running on level and soft surfaces. Ice applied to the area will help to control the problem.

Trauma to the genitalia: Although female athletes can suffer trauma to the reproductive system, those injuries are extremely rare when compared to injuries to the male genitalia. This area has a good supply of blood and nerve endings. A direct blow could cause excruciating pain and temporary disability. A contusion to the testes will produce the same physiological tissue reaction as contusions to other body parts. There is hemorrhaging, fluid effusion, and muscle spasm. One method of relieving this spasm is to have the athlete lie on the ground and flex his thighs to his chest. A cold pack should be applied to the area.

The Hip Pointer: Some of the muscles that control trunk movement attach to the anterior iliac crest. There is little natural protection over this area. Because of this, the muscles can be bruised from a direct blow, such as from a football helmet, from a kick, knee, or elbow, or from falling on the floor. If the force is severe, the muscles can be pinched against the crest of the ilium and bruising or shearing can take place. This injury is called a hip pointer and it can range from mild to severe. With all hip pointers, there is immediate pain; swelling may or may not be present. Any movement requiring involvement of the trunk will result in more pain. Severe hip pointers are quite limiting because of the common functions of the damaged muscles.

Hip dislocation: A hip dislocation is a dangerous condition that should only be handled by emergency medical personnel. In most cases, the athlete will be lying on his or her back. The leg on the injured side will be flexed and externally rotated. Never attempt to reduce such a dislocation. Nerves and blood vessels could become permanently damaged by the head of the femur.

Rehabilitation

Sending an athlete back to competition before healing is complete leaves the player susceptible to further injury. The best way to determine when healing is complete is by the absence of pain during stressful activity and by the return of pain free full range of motion and strength.

Prior to the beginning of any rehabilitation exercise program, the athletic trainer should consult with a medical doctor to establish a program tailored for that individual athlete and the specific injury to be rehabilitated. The following exercises can be used as preventive or rehabilitative exercises:

Hip and Pelvis:
- Hip Flexion
- Hip Extension
- Hip Adduction
- Hip Abduction
- Hip Internal Rotation
- Hip External Rotation

- Squats
- Swimming
- Stationary Bicycle
- Progressive Running Program
- Sport Specific Exercises

Included in any rehabilitation protocol would be the following:
- Range-of-Motion Exercises
- Resistance Exercises
- Sport Specific Exercises

<u>Preventive/Supportive Techniques</u>

Taping is a time-honored and time-consuming tradition. It is also a very expensive practice. Whether to tape healthy body parts is a decision the athletic trainer will have to make.

All injured joints should be taped initially. The purpose of taping is to keep the joint from moving so the ligaments won't be stretched further. Listed below is a review of techniques that are outlined in *The Comprehensive Manual of Taping and Wrapping Techniques* published by Cramer Products.

Hip and Pelvic:
- Hip Flexor Wrap
- Hip Adductor Wrap
- Hip Pointer Taping

NATA Competency Terms

Listed below is a list of musculoskeletal conditions/disorders that affect the hip and pelvis. A valuable learning experience would be to define and review these conditions in a medical dictionary and/or sports medicine textbook.

- Contusions of the Thigh (1, 2, 3 degree)
- Dislocation
- Fracture (pelvis or femur)

- Iliac Crest Contusion (Hip Pointer)
- Iliotibial Band Syndrome
- Myositis Ossificians

- Sprain
- Strain
- Tendinitis

Chapter 8 - Review Questions

Completion:

1. It is important to determine muscle _____ and _____ during an injury assessment.

2. When conducting compression tests for the hip apply forces _____/_____ and _____/_____.

3. The muscles of the groin are the _____, the _____ group and the _____ _____ _____.

4. A _____ is the bruising and destruction of soft tissue cells as a result of a direct blow.

5. The hip joint is formed by the spherical head of the _____ fitting into the deep _____ of the hip.

6. Before treating groin strains, _____ _____ must be conducted to identify the injured muscles.

7. The groin muscles control hip flexion and _____ of the leg.

8. The _____ joint is the strongest in the body.

Short Answer:

1. Why are there few injuries involving the hip?

2. What type of joint is the hip?

3. What are the signs of a fracture?

4. What do functional tests include?

5. Why are pelvic fractures rare?

6. Why should you never attempt to reduce a dislocation of the hip?

7. What is the best way to determine when healing is complete?

8. What are the exercises used in prevention/rehabilitation of a hip injury?

9. What are the forms of preventive/supportive wrapping techniques for the hip and pelvis?

10. Explain why the hip joint is the strongest in the body.

11. What complications can occur if a thigh contusion is mishandled?

12. What muscles are most often injured in a groin strain? How is this type of injury handled?

13. What rehabilitation exercises may be done to return an athlete who has suffered a thigh or hip injury back to full sports participation?

NOTES

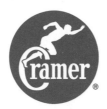

Chapter 9

Thorax And Abdomen Evaluation

Educational Objectives

The learner should, at the completion of the chapter, be able to perform the following:

- Recognize the anatomical structures in the thorax and abdomen.
- Understand the importance of performing the primary survey.
- Recognize the importance of the physical examination.
- Identify the special tests used to determine injury to the area.
- Understand the rehabilitation protocol for this region of the body.
- Recognize the principles involved with taping and wrapping to this section of the body.

Evaluation Format

Fortunately, thoracic and abdominal injuries are less common than extremity injuries. However, these injuries can be life-threatening; therefore, in order to provide appropriate care, these injuries demand immediate evaluation and subsequent activation of the emergency medical system. This chapter outlines general evaluation procedures used to assess thoracic and abdomen injuries. Anatomical components of the thorax and abdomen, their function, specific conditions involving them, and the signs and symptoms usually revealed through evaluation are also presented. Common principles are shared and tests are demonstrated that can aid you, as an examiner, to better assess both acute trauma and non-traumatic conditions.

When thoracic injury is suspected, begin your evaluation with the **PRIMARY SURVEY**. The primary survey assesses:

- **Airway**
- **Breathing**
- **Circulation**

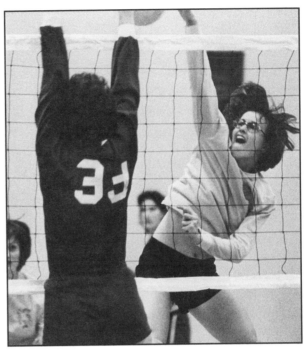

To conduct the primary survey, approach your athlete in a calm and reassuring manner. This enhances relaxation and maintenance of the respiratory and circulatory systems. With the primary survey, be prepared to clear and maintain the airway free of potential obstructions such as blood, vomitus, and foreign matter. Assist the patient in finding the most comfortable position for breathing. Be prepared to provide artificial ventilation or cardiopulmonary resuscitation, CPR, if necessary. If the athlete is unstable, activate the emergency medical system.

Once your primary survey is completed and you determine the athlete's condition is **not** life-threatening, perform a secondary survey. The **secondary survey** consists of two elements—History and Physical Examination. The **History** is that part of the evaluation in which the examiner questions the athlete to determine:

- Mechanism of injury
- Onset of symptoms
- Location of injury
- Quantity and quality of pain
- Type and location of any abnormal sensations
- Progression of signs and symptoms
- Activities that make the symptoms better or worse
- Nausea

- Weakness
- Dyspnea (shortness of breath)

The **Physical Examination** is your next step. Remember, physical examination findings may vary tremendously from athlete to athlete, yet still be within a normal range. Factors such as physical activity and exercise may account for this variance. Some signs and symptoms that may vary are:
- Respiratory rate
- Moistness, color and temperature of skin
- Pulse rate

Essential to the physical examination is the evaluation of **VITAL SIGNS**:
- Abnormal nerve response
- Blood pressure
- Movement
- Pulse
- Pupils
- Respiration
- Skin color
- State of consciousness
- Temperature

Following determination of the vital signs, the Physical Examination then progresses to:
- **Inspection**
- **Auscultation (listening for sounds)**
- **Percussion (tapping)**
- **Palpation And Special Tests**

During the Inspection stage of your physical examination, observe the following:
- Level of consciousness
- Skin color
- The athlete's positions, movements and signs of guarding or apprehension
- Respiratory rate and rhythm for dyspnea (shortness of breath)
- Symmetry of chest appearance and chest movements
- Signs of trauma such as:
  Hemoptysis (coughing up blood)
  Hematemesis (vomiting up blood)

Ecchymosis (escaping of blood into tissue)
- Signs of respiratory distress such as cyanosis (pale or bluish skin color of the lips, fingertips, or fingernails from poor oxygenation of the blood)
- Pupil equality and responsiveness
- Evidence of penetrating trauma
- Vomiting

Next, **Auscultation** is the process of listening for sounds produced in the thoracic and abdominal cavities. A stethoscope is usually used and auscultation is normally conducted by medical professionals with extensive training and experience in this complex skill. The specific techniques of auscultation are beyond the scope of this text. Auscultation determines:
- Normal vs. abnormal chest sounds
- Breathing equality
- Depth of breaths

After completing auscultation, trained medical professionals usually perform percussion. Percussion involves tapping on various parts of the body and noting the sound produced. Percussion assists in determining the presence or absence of certain conditions. For percussion to yield informative results, extensive training and practice are required. Primarily, during percussion, medical professionals:
- Listen for normal/abnormal sounds such as tympany, dullness, or hyperresonance

Palpation and Special Test
Palpation determines:
- General and specific areas of tenderness
- Location of deformities
- Location and extent of swelling
- Air crepitus (produced by air caught in subcutaneous tissue)
- Bony crepitus (produced by the rough edges of fractured bones rubbing together)
- Asymmetry
- Muscle rigidity
- Abdominal rebound tenderness

Special Tests help:

- Evaluate active range of motion
- Provide resistance to movement in the different planes to elicit painful ranges, limitations and musculoskeletal weaknesses
- Evaluate pain and dysfunction associated with inspiration and expiration
- Apply passive stress on the rib cage and sternum to check for fractures/separations

When evaluating **Range of Motion**, your assessment is divided into active, passive, and resistive motions and may be approached from the three cardinal planes of motion, the **Sagittal Plane**, the **Transverse Plane**, and the **Frontal Plane**. Visually note any apprehension, limited range, and painful arcs within each plane. While observing the range of motion, ask the athlete to state and describe the locations and qualities of any abnormal or painful sensations elicited by their movements.

The **Sagittal Plane range of motion test** assesses range of motion limitations and associated findings in the sagittal plane. To evaluate sagittal plane range of motion, the patient stands and slowly flexes the trunk to the point where the hands touch the toes or the floor. Ask the athlete to slowly return from full trunk flexion to trunk extension. The **Transverse Plane range of motion test** assesses range of motion limitations and associated findings in the transverse plane. To evaluate transverse plane range of motion, the athlete stands and slowly rotates the trunk to the right as far as possible. This position is held and then slowly rotated to the extreme left. The **Frontal Plane range of motion test** assesses range of motion limitations and associated findings in the frontal plane. To evaluate frontal plane range of motion, the athlete should stand and slowly, laterally flex the trunk to the right as far as possible. Then the athlete laterally flexes the trunk through the neutral standing position to the far left.

The **Inspiration and Expiration Tests** assess inspiratory and expiratory function and elicit signs and symptoms of thoracic injury. Evaluate **Inspiration and Expiration** by having the athlete breathe in as much air as possible and hold for a few seconds. Then, ask the athlete to breathe out slowly and fully in an attempt to expire all air from the lungs. Instruct the patient to hold the maximally expired position for a few seconds. During these breathing activities, observe any patient apprehension or limitations in the inspiratory movement as well as any display of associated pain. Question the patient regarding location and nature of any symptoms elicited by these procedures. Some specific signs or symptoms are:

- Inability to fully inspire
- Pain during breathing
- Guarding or apprehension with respirations

Next, in assessing thoracic injuries, fractures and separations may occur in the bones and costal cartilages of the rib cage. If there is a complete separation or fracture, crepitus, grating, and popping sensations may be present with active and passive chest movements. In some cases passive stress may be applied to the rib cage to elicit and further appreciate these signs and symptoms. Again, use caution when examining the thorax as other associated internal injuries may exist.

Two tests are performed to determine if rib cage and sternum fractures or separations exist. These chest compression tests are the **Anterior/Posterior Chest Compression Test** and the **Lateral Chest Compression Test**. These chest compression tests can help distinguish between muscle contusions/strains and loss of bony stability and integrity. The chest compression testing may be accomplished in the standing or sitting position. However, if the athlete is having complications, the supine and sidelying position may allow for better patient comfort and relaxation.

Anterior/Posterior Chest Compression Test assesses lateral rib cage bony integrity. To perform the anterior/posterior compression test, instruct the athlete to either sit or stand. You should place the palmar surface of one hand anteriorly on the chest wall at the level of the affected area. Place your other hand at the corresponding level posteriorly.

Compress the rib cage by pushing your hands toward each other. This inward pressure anteriorly and posteriorly will cause the rib cage to bow outward laterally which will elicit pain and bony crepitis if the injury to the lateral rib cage is a fracture. However, if the injury is a contusion or muscle spasm, no pain or crepitis will be elicited.

The Lateral Chest Compression Test assesses anterior or posterior rib cage bony integrity.
To perform the lateral compression test, instruct the patient to either sit or stand. Then, as the examiner, place the palmar surface of your hands laterally on the athlete's chest wall sides at the affected area level. Compress the rib cage by pushing your hands toward each other. This inward pressure from both sides will cause the rib cage to bow outward anteriorly and posteriorly. This inward pressure laterally will cause the rib cage to bow outward which will elicit pain and bony crepitis if the injury to the anterior/posterior lateral rib cage is a fracture. However, if the injury is a contusion or muscle spasm, no pain or crepitis will be elicited.

Thorax Anatomy and Common Injuries

Now let's look closely at some anatomical components of the **Thorax**: their functions, specific conditions involving them, and the signs and symptoms usually revealed through evaluation. A brief presentation on how the thorax may be managed by medical personnel is presented. Acute traumatic injuries occurring to the **Thorax** may involve the heart, lungs, and rib cage. Remember, evaluation of such injuries require current First Aid and C.P.R. certification. As an allied health professional, it is essential that you are trained in current basic life support techniques.

The **Heart** is located in the center of the thoracic cavity and positioned slightly to the left. It pumps oxygenated blood from the heart to the body and de-oxygenated blood from itself to the lungs. One of the more common conditions involving the heart is a myocardial infarction, commonly referred to as a heart attack. **Myocardial infarction** is ischemia (decrease in oxygenated blood flow) to cardiac tissue which may result in a disturbance of normal heart function characterized by arrhythmia.

86

Signs and Symptoms of Myocardial Infarction are:
- Persistent chest pain or pressure unrelieved by rest, position changes, or medication

- Breathing difficulty: noisier, shorter, faster than normal
- Irregular pulse rate: faster or slower than normal
- Cyanosis
- Moist face or profuse sweating
- Radiation of pain to the left side (neck, shoulder, arm)
- Levine's sign (clenched fist over the chest)
- Hypotension or shock

As an allied health professional you should be aware of other conditions involving the heart including cardiac contusions and pericardial tamponade (compression of the heart). These conditions occur quite rarely but the results can be catastrophic, particularly if they are not immediately recognized and appropriately managed. **Cardiac contusions** result from a direct blow to the anterior chest wall in the heart region. Blunt trauma to the anterior chest wall may cause pericardial tamponade. With **pericardial tamponade**, bleeding accumulates inside the pericardial sac and will gradually increase, causing external pressure on the heart, thereby preventing proper contraction.

The Lungs, located in the thoracic cavity and protected by the rib cage, are formed by a network of branching tubes and air sacs. This network provides respiration whereby the blood from the body is re-oxygenated. A **Pneumothorax** occurs either spontaneously or traumatically from blunt or sharp trauma to the chest wall. Pneumothorax is characterized by air accumulation in the pleural space. The air escapes from the lung upon each inspiration, collects in the pleural space and eventually results in lung collapse. **Spontaneous, traumatic**, and tension pneumothorax signs and symptoms should be explored with your patient. Spontaneous pneumothorax may occur suddenly without trauma as a result of weakness in the lung wall. A **Traumatic pneumothorax** will occur as a result of accumulation of air in the pleural space due to trauma. One or both lungs may be involved.

A **Tension pneumothorax** may result when the air escaping from the lung enters the pleural cavity and is not allowed to return to the lung due to the one-way valve created in the lung wall. This trapping of air in the pleural cavity causes intrapleural pressure to increase and progressively compromises venous return and further ventilation by pushing structures to the contralateral side.

A **Hemothorax** is similar to a pneumothorax, however, blood, instead of air, collects in the pleural cavity. A Hemothorax occurs from bleeding caused by fractured ribs or other trauma. If it occurs in conjunction with a pneumothorax it is referred to as a **Hemopneumothorax**. **Pulmonary contusion** is caused by a direct blow to the chest, producing bruising to the lungs. As with any bruise, blood vessels are injured and a considerable amount of blood escapes into the lung tissue.

Thoracic related bony and joint injuries can occur to the rib cage structure. The **Rib Cage** outlines the thoracic borders and provides protection to the heart, lungs, great vessels (aorta and vena cava), liver, and spleen. Its ability to expand and relax is essential in assisting the lungs' respiratory function. Other than contusions and strains, **rib fractures** are the most common injuries seen in the thoracic area. Nondisplaced fractures are usually benign; however, displaced fractures may result in lacerations to the lung and associated intercostal vessels. You should remember the following about rib fractures:

- **Non-displaced are the most common**
- **Displaced rib fractures may result in laceration of the lung or an associated intercostal vessel**
- **Injuries usually involve the 5th to 9th ribs**
- **Tremendous forces are necessary to fracture the 1st and 2nd ribs**
- **Fracture of 7th through 12th ribs may be associated with liver, spleen, or kidney injuries**

The signs and symptoms of rib fractures are:
- Pain at fracture site aggravated by coughing, breathing, movement, and compression tests
- Dyspnea (shortness of breath)
- Localized tenderness
- Bony or air crepitation
- Contusion
- Ecchymosis (escaping of blood into tissue)

Sternal Fractures are rare but may occur from high-impact injuries. The signs and symptoms are:
- Pain directly over sternum
- Pain aggravated by deep inspiration
- Possible associated myocardial contusion

Costochondral sprains and **separations** result from twisting injuries or blows to the anterolateral chest. Costochondral sprains are most common in contact sports and generally elicit joint soreness and stiffness. In a costochondral separation, disrupted cartilage and bone override each other, causing localized sharp pain followed by intermittent stabbing pain.

Signs and Symptoms are:
- Tenderness over costochondral junction
- Deformity due to displacement
- Pain with inspiration, expiration or compression test

Sternoclavicular seperations may occur from falls on the acromioclavicular joint or from lateral blows to the glenohumeral joint, which transmit force through the clavicle to the sternoclavicular joint. Anterior dislocation is most common. However, posterior dislocations produce life-threatening impingement on airway or great vessels.

Signs and symptoms are:
- Proximal clavicle may displace anteriorly, superiorly, or posteriorly
- Pain, swelling, and noticeable displacement of sternoclavicular joint

A **Flail chest** is often a life-threatening injury which results when several ribs are fractured in two places.

Although all injuries to the thoracic cavity can be life-threatening, some injuries are classified non-life threatening. When evaluating, you will generally find that most of these injuries are caused by either a direct blow or stretching of the soft tissue. **Rib contusions** are one category of musculoskeletal related non-life threatening injuries, but are quite common and result from direct contact to the rib cage.

Signs and symptoms are:

- Point tenderness
- Possible ecchymosis
- Pain with excessive movement
- Pain with deep inspiration/expiration
- Lack of crepitus
- Negative compression test

Muscular strains result when the tensile force placed on a muscle exceeds its contraction capabilities, thereby causing structural damage to the muscle fibers. Signs and symptoms could include:

- Point tenderness to direct palpation
- Pain with contractile movements of involved muscle
- Pain with passive stretching of involved muscle
- Weakness in movements controlled by involved muscle
- Deformity of muscle on the chest
- Ecchymosis
- Negative compression test

Muscle tears to the pectoralis major muscle usually result when a violent contraction against a heavy resistance occurs. **Rupture of the pectoralis** major would display these symptoms:

- Sudden, sharp pain in upper arm or chest
- Ecchymosis
- Weakened adduction, flexion, internal rotation
- Deformity of muscle on the chest
- Muscular defect may be evident in axillary fold

There are other conditions related to the thoracic cavity, which, as a health professional, you should be aware of and learn more about. **Respiratory** conditions related to the thoracic cavity are common. Following are some conditions and brief definitions.

Asthma—An inflammatory respiratory condition characterized by bronchospasm (wheezing) and shortness of breath (dyspnea). Asthma may be exercise induced.

Bronchitis—Inflammation of the bronchial tubes. Bronchitis is usually characterized by a progressive cough.

Hemoptysis—Expectoration of blood arising from the lungs (patient's coughing up blood or blood-stained sputum).

Hyperventilation—Increase in respiratory rate usually associated with anxiety which causes a change in the acid-base balance of the blood. Symptoms include dyspnea and numbness and tingling in the hands, fingers, and around the mouth.

Influenza—A viral illness characterized as an acute onset of fatigue, muscle ache, headache, and fever; usually lasts one to two weeks.

Pleuritic chest wall pain—Inflammation of the serous membrane lining, which lies between the lung and chest wall, causing pain with inspiration and expiration or cough.

Pneumonia—Inflammation of the lungs caused primarily by bacteria, viruses, chemical irritants, vegetable dusts, and allergy. Usual symptoms are fever, cough, and chest pain.

Others disorders of the **Circulatory** system include **Tachycardia**, **Bradycardia**, and **Arrhythmia**.

Tachycardia— Abnormal rapidity of heart action and usually defined in adults as a heart rate over 100 beats per minute.

Bradycardia— Abnormal slowness of heart action and usually defined in adults as a heart rate under 60 beats per minute.

Arrhythmia— Abnormal heart rhythm characterized by skipping of beat or an irregular pulse.

Immediate Referral is necessary if the following signs and symptoms are present in a thoracic assessment.

- **Difficulty in breathing**
- **Shortness of breath—inability to catch breath**
- **Severe pain increasing in chest**
- **Vomiting or coughing up blood**
- **Diminished chest movement on the affected side**
- **Shifting or moving of trachea with each breath**
- **Suspected rib fracture or costochondral separation**
- **Signs of shock**
- **Doubt regarding the nature and severity of the chest injury**

Abdomen Anatomy and Common Injuries

The abdominal cavity is divided into the four quadrants: Right Upper, Left Upper, Right Lower and Left Lower. Organs most commonly affected by injury or conditions will be outlined in this chapter. However, you should be familiar with the anatomical location of each organ in specific quadrants and their function.

Major organs of the **Right Upper** quadrant included are liver, gallbladder, right kidney and adrenal gland, pylorus of the stomach, head of pancreas, portion of colon, and small intestine. Major organs of the **Left Upper** quadrant included are stomach, spleen, left kidney and adrenal gland, portion of the pancreas, portion of the colon, and small intestine. Major organs in the **Right Lower** quadrant included are appendix, portion of the small and large intestines, portion of the colon, and structures of the urinary and reproductive systems. A portion of the small and large intestine, portion of the colon, and structures of the urinary and reproductive system are located in the **Left Lower** quadrant.

When examining the abdomen, each quadrant should be auscultated, percussed, and palpated. The **Valsalva Maneuver** is used to provoke an increase in pain or mass protrusion if significant intra-abdominal trauma has occurred. To perform the Valsalva maneuver, have the athlete take a deep breath and then close his or her airway and strain as if having a bowel movement. Any worsening of pain or mass protrusion through the abdominal wall is considered a positive test. The **Iliopsoas Test** and **Obsturator Test** detect the possibility of peritoneal irritation. The **Heel Pound Test** may also detect the possibility of peritoneal irritation.

Now let's look closely at some anatomical components of the abdomen, their functions, specific conditions involving them, and the signs and symptoms usually revealed through evaluation. We will briefly show how they may appear upon presentation and how they may need to be managed by medical personnel. Acute traumatic injuries involving the abdomen may occur to the:

Hollow Organs
- Stomach
- Gall bladder
- Urinary bladder
- Intestines
- Vessels

Solid Organs
- Spleen
- Liver
- Kidneys
- Abdominal Muscles

Hollow Organs

The **Stomach** is J-shaped and found directly underneath the diaphragm in the left upper abdominal quadrant. The stomach receives food from the esophagus and begins the digestive process. The **Small Intestine** is principally located in the left and right lower quadrants but has portions in both upper quadrants. Its major functions are digestion and absorption. The **Large Intestine** is an inverted, U-shaped organ that is located in all quadrants and functions in completing the absorption process and in the formation and removal of waste products. The key to successful management of **hollow organ** injury is rapid detection through evaluation and control of hemorrhage and abdominal contamination. The signs and symptoms of hollow organs injury are:
- Decreased bowel sounds
- Tender abdomen
- Hard or rigid abdomen
- Guarding
- Distended abdomen
- Signs and symptoms of shock—hypotension and tachycardia

The **Spleen** is the body's largest lymphatic organ and is located in the left upper quadrant, directly below the diaphragm and behind the 9th, 10th, and 11th ribs. It serves as a reservoir of red blood cells and regulates the number of red blood cells in circulation. The spleen also destroys old or defective

red blood cells and produces white blood cells. Signs and symptoms of spleen injury are:
- Signs of acute abdominal pain
- **Rebound tenderness**
- **Rigidity**
- **Guarding**
- Abdominal pain in left upper quadrant
- Left shoulder or neck pain (Kehr's Sign)
- Shock
- Possible rib fracture

The **Liver** is located in the right upper quadrant with a small portion found in the left upper quadrant. It is a solid organ with a variety of functions including manufacturing of plasma proteins, manufacturing and storage of blood cells, removal of old or defective red blood cells, breakdown of toxic substance, glucose and fat metabolism, mineral and vitamin storage, and bile production. Signs and symptoms of acute liver injury are:
- Signs of acute abdominal pain
- **Rebound tenderness**
- **Rigidity**
- **Guarding**
- Abdominal pain in right upper quadrant
- Right shoulder or neck pain
- Possible right, lower rib fracture

The **Kidneys** are paired solid, bean-shaped organs located in both the right and left upper quadrants near the spine. The Kidneys function to help control blood volume. They also remove waste from the blood in the form of urine. Signs and symptoms of kidney injury are:
- Signs of acute abdominal pain
- **Rebound tenderness**
- **Rigidity**
- **Guarding**
- Hematuria (passing of blood in urine)
- Bloody discharge or inability to void
- Flank or low back pain
- Positive Grey-Turner sign—ecchymosis in flank
- No acute abdominal signs
- Possible bony crepitus due to rib fracture

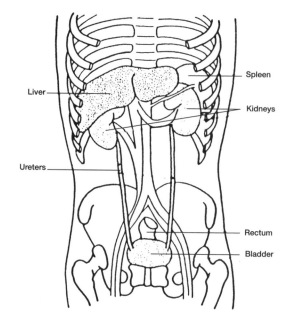

*The abdominal organs (source: **Modern Principles of Athletic Training**, 5th Ed., Daniel D. Arnheim, 1985.)*

In examining the **Abdominal Muscles**, the **Rectus Abdominis** runs vertically from the xiphoid process and the costal cartilages of the 5th, 6th, and 7th ribs to the crest of the pubis. In addition to providing protection of the abdominal contents, the rectus abdominis flexes, laterally flexes, and rotates the trunk. The **External Obliques** run in a superolateral to inferomedial direction from the borders of the eight lower ribs to insert on the anterior crest of the ilium and pubis as well as the rectus abdominis fascia. Vital in protecting the abdomen, these muscles also assist in flexion and are heavily involved in trunk rotation. The **Internal Obliques** run in an inferolateral to superomedial direction from the anterior two-thirds of the iliac crest and lumbar fascia to insert on the costal cartilages of the 8th, 9th, and 10th ribs and the linea alba. In addition to abdominal protection, these muscles assist in flexion and are heavily involved in trunk rotation.

Muscular strains result when the tensile forces placed on a muscle exceed its contraction capabilities, thereby causing muscular fiber structural damage. Contusions result from direct blows to the abdominal wall. Signs and symptoms of abdominal injury are:

- Superficial, but not deep tenderness to palpation
- Point tenderness to direct palpation
- Pain with contractile movements of involved muscle
- Pain with passive stretching of involved muscle
- Weakness in movements controlled by involved muscle
- Deformity of muscle
- Ecchymosis
- Positive bowel sounds
- No distention
- No signs and symptoms of shock

Hematomas may develop from strains but more commonly result from contusions.

Although all abdominal injuries can be life-threatening, some are classified as non-traumatic. **Non-traumatic injuries/conditions of the abdomen include:**

Appendicitis—Inflammation of the appendix. Generally affects the young and is more common in males. Appendicitis is characterized by high fever, abdominal pain often localized in the right lower quadrant, nausea, vomiting, and anorexia. May have signs of acute abdomen pain.

Dysmenorrhea—Pain associated with menstruation.

Ectopic pregnancy—Implantation of the fertilized ovum outside of the uterine cavity.

Gastroenteritis—Inflammation of the stomach and intestinal tract. Characterized by one or more of the following symptoms: nausea, vomiting, diarrhea. Usually due to viral infection, but can be bacterially induced.

Hernia—Protrusion of abdominal viscera through a portion of the abdominal wall.

Indigestion (heartburn)—Incomplete or imperfect digestion, usually accompanied by one or more of the following symptoms: pain, nausea, vomiting.

Stitch in the side (sideache)—Sharp pain in the side usually associated with strenuous physical activity. May be caused by muscle spasm and/or trapped gas.

Immediate Referral is necessary if the following signs and symptoms are revealed in an abdominal assessment:

- Signs of acute abdominal pain
- **Rebound tenderness**
- **Rigidity**
- **Guarding**
- Signs of shock
- Blood in the urine or stool
- Prolonged discomfort, sensation of weakness, or pulling in groin
- Superficial protrusion or palpable mass
- Increasing nausea
- Vomiting
- Doubt regarding the nature and severity of the abdominal injury
- Presence of fever
- Severe abdominal pain
- Presence of radiating or referred pain

Rehabilitation

Prior to initiating a rehabilitative program, a proper evaluation must be completed. All injuries should be thoroughly evaluated by a physician or athletic trainer with recommendations concerning proper treatment and rehabilitative exercises outlined. Listed below are types of exercises for each joint.

Exercises for the Thorax:
- Pectoral butterflies
- Pectoral stretching
- Arm extension stretches

Exercises for the Abdomen:
- Abdominal crunches
- Oblique abdominal crunches
- Modified push ups with pelvis stabilized to stretch abdomen

Preventive/Supportive Techniques

Listed below is a overview of taping and wrapping techniques outlined in the textbook titled *The Comprehensive Manual of Taping and Wrapping Techniques* produced by Cramer Products. Please review this text for complete directions on how to apply these preventive/supportive techniques.

- Low Back Taping
- Rib Taping
- Hip Flexor Wrap
- Adductor Wrap
- Hip Pointer Taping
- Acromioclavicular Joint Taping
- Glenohumeral Joint Taping

Chapter 9 - Review Questions

Completion:

1. The _____ _____ is the beginning of a suspected thoracic injury evaluation.

2. _____/_____ _____ test and _____ _____ test can differentiate between a contusion/muscle spasm injury and possible rib fracture.

3. Inflammation of the peritoneum that lines the abdominal cavity is usually called _____ .

4. A myocardial infarction is commonly referred to as a _____ _____ .

5. A heart rate over 100 beats per minute in adults is commonly a disorder known as _____ .

6. Traumatic injuries to the thorax may involve the _____ , _____ , and _____ .

7. A _____ _____ is often a life threatening injury which results when several ribs are fractured in two places.

Short Answer:

1. Name two important organs in the thoracic cavity.
-
-

2. Define the two respiratory conditions found in many athletes.
-
-

3. Name the four quadrants of the abdominal cavity and a specific organ of concern in each.
-
-
-
-

4. What are the four vital signs?
-
-
-
-

5. Name two supportive techniques for the thoracic cavity.
-
-

6. What are the three elements for auscultation assessment?
-
-
-

7. Acute traumatic injuries occurring to the thorax may involve what three elements?
-
-
-

8. Name the signs of acute abdominal injury.

9. List the suggested rehabilitation for the thorax.

10. List the suggested rehabilitation for the abdomen.

11. Name the suggested textbook for taping and wrapping.

12. What is the primary survey for a thoracic injury?

13. What does the secondary survey consist of?

13. How many quadrants are there in the abdomen?

14. What are the signs and symptoms that are revealed in your abdominal assessment for immediate referral?

15. What are the signs and symptoms of myocardial infarction?

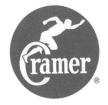

NOTES

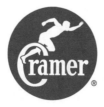

Chapter 10

The Head, Neck, and Spine

Educational Objectives

The learner should, at the completion of the chapter, be able to perform the following:

- Understand the anatomy of the head, neck, and spine.
- Recognize the importance of the proper evaluation of injuries to this region of the body.
- Identify the common injuries associated with the head, neck, and spine.
- Understand the protocol for rehabilitation exercises of this region.
- Identify the NATA competencies for this section of the body.

Student athletic trainers are not responsible for stabilizing or transporting severely injured athletes. The student athletic trainer's responsibilities in emergency situations include becoming aware of the causes of serious injuries, making sure equipment and the playing area are safe, recognizing signs of serious injury and alerting the coach and team physician of these dangers, and making sure the school has a detailed plan to handle emergency transport.

Anatomy

For our purposes, we will consider the head in two parts: the cranium, which encases the brain, and the face. The brain is protected from trauma by the bones of the skull. Other bones of the head include the mandible, or jaw, and the bones of the face. The head has the best blood supply of the body.

Seven cervical vertebra makeup the bones of the neck. The cervical spine, with its attached ligaments and muscles, is adequate to support the head, which weighs about fourteen pounds. Other structures in the neck are the larynx, trachea, muscles,

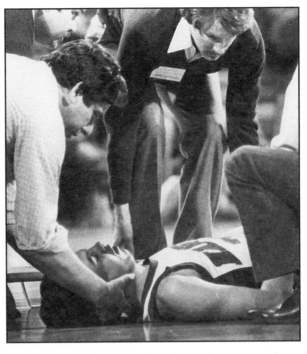

nerves, and blood vessels. The neck is a very fragile region of the body, in which injuries can occur to the seven cervical vertebrae. The cervical section of the spine is by far the most flexible, allowing flexion, extension and rotation of the neck and head.

The neck is seldom injured in daily activities, including sports. However, those injuries that do occur to the neck have the potential to cause paralysis and even death. This is because the vertebrae, like other bones, can be fractured or sprained. Without protection of the vertebrae in their correct alignment, permanent spinal cord damage can occur. The spinal cord transmits impulses that control all voluntary and involuntary movements of the body.

Muscles allow the head, neck, and spine to move in different movement patterns. Listed below is a brief outline of the anatomy of the head, neck and spine:

Head and Neck - Bones:

- Cranial Bones
- Vertebral Column
- Cervical (7)
- Thoracis (12)
- Lumbar (5)
- Sacral (5)
- Coccyx (4 fused)

Neck and Spine - Muscles:

- Sternocleidomastoidius
- Trapezius
- Levator scapulae
- Deltoid
- Coracobrachialis
- Teres major
- Latissimus dorsi
- Supraspinatus
- Subscapularis
- Pectoralis major
- Erector spinae

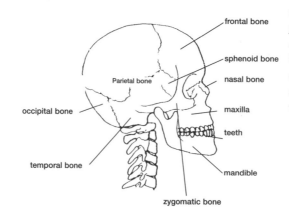

The bones of the skull protect the brain from trauma. However, a forceful blow to rthe head can cause a concussion, or shaking of the brain within the skull.

Head and Neck - Movement:

- Flexion (touch chin to chest)
- Extension (look directly at the ceiling)
- Rotation (move head in circular pattern)
- Lateral bending
- Protraction
- Retraction
- Elevation
- Depression

Spine - Movement:

- Flexion
- Extension
- Lateral Bending
- Rotation

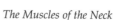

The Muscles of the Neck

Evaluation of Head Injuries

The athlete sustaining a head injury may recover from the initial trauma and have all signs of recovery, and then suddenly show signs of deteriorating conditions. If the arteries surrounding the brain have been torn, signs and symptoms may be present within minutes, while rupturing of veins may not produce symptoms for days. Therefore, <u>any athlete sustaining a head injury should be monitored a minimum of 24 hours and carefully evaluated on a regular basis for at least one week.</u> Brain injury as a result of external trauma can be classified into three primary categories of intracranial hemorrhaging: epidural, subdural, and intracerebral.

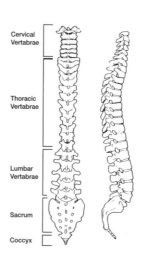

The Vertebrae can be fractured or dislocated, just like any other bone. Because the vertebrae column encases the spinal cord, any injury to the vertebrae can result in permanent paralysis or death.

Epidural—If the arteries located in the dural membrane are torn, a hematoma (blood clot) will rapidly accumulate, usually in a specific area, due to the epidural covering lying in close association to the skull. The athlete who shows all signs of recovery (the "lucid interval") soon demonstrates signs of a serious head injury.

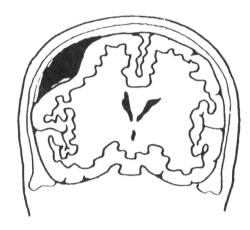

When the brain is traumatized, there is internal bleeding. However, unlike other areas of the body, the brain has very little room to swell. This can result in epidural bleeding.

Subdural—When the veins connecting the dura-matter to the brain are ruptured, hemorrhaging may spread over a much greater area and, therefore, signs may develop at a much slower rate. It may takes hours or days to develop symptoms of brain damage.

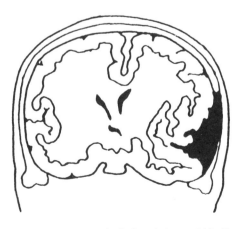

When the brain is traumatized, there is internal bleeding. However, unlike other areas of the body, the brain has very little room to swell. This can result in subdural bleeding.

Intracerebral—Bleeding within the brain usually has a fast onset and will require immediate hospitalization to avoid brain damage.

Secondary conditions may also arise as a result of a head injury. A **Cerebral edema** is localized swelling at the injury site, may be evident within 12 hours, and is characterized by headache and occasional seizures. **Seizures** may occur immediately following a head injury or within a 24-hour period of time. For the athlete having a seizure, be certain that the victim's airway is maintained, he is safe from further harm, and has his head turned to the side to allow saliva and blood to drain. **Migraine headaches** are an attack of severe headaches accompanied by partial blindness in the field of vision and loss of sensation in the limbs and/or face may develop as a result of head injury.

A **Concussion** is defined as a shaking of the brain. Forceful blows to the head, or even to other parts of the body, can cause this shaking. A player does not have to suffer a loss of consciousness to have suffered a concussion. Concussions can occur in football, wrestling, gymnastics, basketball, or any sport where hard contact is made, either with another player, with equipment or with the ground. Even though a single blow can cause a concussion, the accumulated effects of numerous minor blows can also cause a concussion.

When the brain is traumatized, as in a concussion, the body's response will be the same as with other tissue injuries there will be internal hemorrhage. Unlike other areas of the body, though, the brain has very little room to swell because of the encasing skull. Also, this internal hemorrhage is one type of bleeding that can not be controlled with cold, compression, and elevation. Besides the original tissue damage from the concussion, additional damage is possible from the internal hemorrhage, which has no outlet or area in which to expand. This pressure on the brain will affect the central nervous system, causing various reactions in the body. Concussions are classified as **mild, moderate, or severe,** depending on the amount of damage done to the brain. Each classification of injury may produce any or all of the following signs.

1. Mild concussion symptoms: No loss of consciousness, possible loss of memory (temporary), some mental confusion, unsteadiness, ringing in the ears, minor dizziness, dull headache, rapid recovery from all symptoms. The team physician will make the decision whether an athlete who has suffered any concussion, even a mild one, can return to play. Before getting that permission, the athlete must be completely aware of his or her surroundings. Even with a suspected mild concussion, the athlete must be observed for worsening symptoms. It is recommended that no athlete be permitted to participate as long as he or she has a headache or any other symptoms caused by a blow to the head.

2. Moderate concussion symptoms: Loss of consciousness for up to two or three minutes, inability to remember events that occurred before losing consciousness, nausea, dizziness, ringing in the ears, disturbance of balance, frequent headaches after other symptoms have subsided. The athlete should not be permitted to re-enter practice or competition. Immediate physician referral is required. Continuous observation for 24 hours to be aware of worsening symptoms is essential.

3. Severe concussion symptoms: Loss of consciousness for more than two or three minutes (which may result in a coma), lack of response to painful stimuli in the extremities, possible wandering eye movements, severe retrograde amnesia, inequality of pupil size, possible convulsions. An athlete with a severe concussion should be transported to the hospital by emergency personnel. As with all head injuries, the ambulance crew will also assume there is a neck injury. In caring for an athlete who has suffered a concussion, quick action is mandatory. It must be stressed again that the athletic trainer or coach should always suspect that the athlete has suffered a neck injury in addition to the concussion. The athlete should not be moved unless it is necessary to provide an airway while medical help is being summoned.

Regardless of the severity of the concussion, a physician must examine the athlete to determine when activity may be resumed. The coach should obtain a signed statement from the physician before the athlete is allowed to return to activity.

Evaluation Format

The first purpose of an evaluation of head injuries is to determine, to the best of your ability, if there is a fracture, cranial bleeding or a concussion. Initially, a fracture or concussion should always be suspected. Signs of a fracture include, but are not limited to, direct or indirect pain, deformity, or a grating sound at the injury site. Some fractures are not accompanied by swelling or pain. If a fracture is suspected, the evaluation stops and the athlete should be referred immediately to a physician.

The evaluation process to help determine the type of injury involves four steps: history, observation, palpation, and stress tests.

(H) History: This involves asking questions of the athlete to help determine the mechanism of injury. Answers to these questions will help the physician in a diagnosis.

(O) Observation: Look for bleeding, deformity, swelling, discoloration, and scars. The athletic trainer should also look for bleeding or straw colored fluid from the ears or nose. This may be an indication of a serious head injury.

(P) Palpation: Any palpation (physical inspection) of the head should take into account the possibility of bleeding from the scalp and appropriate measures should be taken to prevent the spread of bloodborne pathogens from the injured athlete. Palpate the area away from the injury first, working toward the injury site. The entire area around the injury may be sore, but the athletic trainer should try to pinpoint the site of most severe pain. That will be the site where the most damage has been done. From knowledge of the head, neck, and spine's anatomy, the type and extent of injury can be evaluated. Involve the athlete in the evaluation as much as possible. Asking questions that require specific answers can provide valuable information.

(S) Stress Tests: With all tests, the athletic trainer is looking for pain and instability. Note: It is possible to further damage an injured area through manipulation. Years of training are necessary before an athletic trainer would be considered competent to make stress tests and functional tests. These tests are well beyond the expertise of a student athletic trainer. Functional Tests: To determine if damage has been done to muscles, the athletic trainer uses functional tests, including range of motion. The athlete performs active and resistive exercises through all ranges of motion against the athletic trainer's resistance. Pain or weakness could indicate muscle damage.

Refer to Chapter 2 for a full explanation of the H.O.P.S. injury evaluation format.

Common Injuries

Referral to a physician is critical when serious injury occurs to either the head, neck, and/or spine. If any of these situation exist, immediate referral is critical.

- Unconsciousness
- Paralysis
- Obvious deformity
- Suspected fracture or dislocation
- Pain, tenderness, or deformity along the vertebral column
- Significant swelling and pain
- Loss of sensation (motor or sensory)
- Loss of motion
- Doubt regarding the presence of intracranial bleeding
- Bleeding from ears, mouth, and/or nose

Cervical Fractures and Dislocations

The mechanism of injury is any force that flexes, extends, or rotates the neck beyond its normal range of motion. These movements can occur in any sport, but most neck damage is the result of diving or football injuries. Neck injuries are also possible in gymnastics, wrestling, basketball, and other contact sports. Symptoms of cervical fracture or dislocation include:

- Pain in the cervical region or back
- Muscle spasm
- Swelling
- Inability to move the neck (Don't move the neck to test for pain.)
- Numbness, tingling, or burning sensation in the limbs
- Decreased limb strength
- Paralysis below the site of the fracture
- Deformity in the cervical area
- History of the injury

Any history of forced flexion or hyperextension, whiplash, forced rotation, or a hard head-on blow should alert the athletic trainer or coach to the possibility of a fracture or dislocation of the cervical vertebrae. Prevention of neck injuries depends a great deal on the athlete using safe and proper techniques. Neck strength and flexibility, as well as proper protective equipment, can also help prevent neck injuries. If a cervical injury is suspected, emergency medical help should be summoned. The athlete should be left lying in the same position; sandbags to limit any movement should be placed at strategic locations until qualified medical help arrives. **Never allow removal of a football helmet from a player with a possible neck injury!** Also, remember that it is not necessary for the athlete to have neck pain with a neck injury. Cardiopulmonary resuscitation (CPR) classes are available to provide instruction on maintaining an open airway in emergency situations such as this.

Cervical Nerve Stretch Syndrome (Brachial Plexus)

A cervical injury often seen in football is the stretching of one or more of the brachial plexus nerves. This nerve group begins in the neck and innervates the upper extremities. A common name for this injury is a "burner" or "stinger." When the brachial plexus becomes stretched or contused, a burning sensation is produced that extends from the point of injury into the arm. A temporary loss of function and some numbness of the arm may also result. The mechanism of injury is usually forced lateral movement of the head. An athlete who has suffered from cervical nerve stretch syndrome must be removed from competition and checked by a physician. Even though symptoms may disappear rapidly, an examination is needed to rule out a more serious injury. Written clearance by the physician should be obtained by the coach before further athletic participation is permitted.

Epistaxis (Nosebleed)

Usually the result of a direct blow, a nosebleed is a common, minor injury in athletics. There are many first aid methods that have proved successful in stopping the bleeding quickly. One method is to have the athlete sit up, pinching the affected nostril(s) closed. A cold pack should be held over the nose. The athlete's head should be tilted forward; tilting the head back will cause the blood to drip into the throat. Bleeding should stop within five minutes. If the bleeding does not stop after using this method, the student trainer can apply an astringent to a cotton tipped applicator; the astringent is then dabbed onto the site of hemorrhage. Then, a rolled-up sterile gauze pad can be used to plug the nose. The use of a cold pack should be continued.

Eyeball Contusion

All injuries to the eyes must be taken seriously. If the contusion is severe enough, vision could be affected permanently. Concussions are also a consideration when there is a sharp blow to the eye area. Fortunately, most eye contusions are minor. Capillary bleeding can produce discoloration, or the familiar "black eye." Despite swelling of tissue, the vision remains normal in minor contusions. Signs of more serious contusions include blurred, double or spotty vision, and pain. Blood in the eye is also an indication of serious injury. In such cases, both eyes should be patched to reduce movement, a cold pack should be applied, and the athlete should be taken to a physician for diagnosis. Note: chemical cold packs should never be used around the eyes because of' the danger of the packs leaking.

Foreign Body in the Eye

When a foreign object gets into a person's eye, the natural response is to rub the eye. However, rubbing the eye can cause two problems. First, the object may scratch the eye, creating greater discomfort and damage. Second, the object may become embedded in the tissue of the eye, making it more difficult to remove. In removing a foreign body from the surface of the eye:
• Pull down the lower lid to see if that will uncover the object and remove with sterile gauze.
• If the object is under the upper lid, have the athlete look down, grasp the eyelashes of the upper lid and pull the upper lid forward and down over the lower lid. It is possible that this may dislodge the object.
• If unsuccessful, try flushing the eye with water.
• If none of the above work, apply a protective dressing over both eyes and refer to a physician.

Dental Injuries

Most dental injuries and conditions can be painful or distracting, but do not require emergency treatment. Simple first aid measures should be adequate until the athlete can see a dentist. An interested dentist should be part of each athletic department's sports medicine team. Reviewing first aid and emergency treatment procedures with the dentist in the off-season will help the athletic trainer and coach be prepared for common dental problems.

Dental Fractures

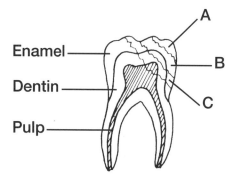

A. Fracture through enamel only
B. Fracture through enamel and dentin
C. Fracture that includes pulp

A mouthpiece will reduce the incidence of concussion and dental injuries by cushioning the teeth from the shock of blows to the jaw. These devices are so effective that their use has all but eliminated dental injuries in football. Athletes in other contact sports, such as basketball and field hockey, could also benefit from wearing protective mouthguards. Mouthpieces should be comfortable so athletes will wear them, and the coach or student athletic trainer should inspect them regularly for wear. Worn mouthpieces must be replaced immediately to help prevent dental injuries.

Back Injuries

The most common back injuries are minor strains, sprains and contusions. These injuries are often caused by sudden or forceful twisting, a direct blow, improper mechanics, or a lack of flexibility. If an injury this serious is suspected, the athlete should not be moved except by an ambulance crew. Remember, a fracture to the vertebra can occur. Mishandling of a vertebral fracture can cause spinal cord damage, resulting in paralysis.

One of the most frustrating and nagging problems in athletics is back strain. There are very few movements in sports that do not use the muscles of the back in some degree of extension, lateral flexion, rotation, or in stretching, as in flexing the trunk. When the back muscles are strained, all of the movements that we have just mentioned will produce some degree of discomfort in the athlete. Even the maintenance of normal posture can be uncomfortable. Any injury to the back should be treated conservatively.

Rehabilitation

Prior to initiating a rehabilitation program, a proper evaluation must be completed. All injuries should be thoroughly evaluated by a physician or athletic trainer with recommendations concerning proper treatment and rehabilitative exercises outlined. The following components should be incorporated in a comprehensive rehabilitation program: full range of motion; pain-free activity; strength, power, and endurance to muscles surrounding joint; and total body conditioning. Listed below are types of rehabilitation exercises for each joint.

Cervical:
- Neck flexion
- Neck extension
- Neck sidebending
- Neck rotation
- Scapular retraction
- Shoulder shrugs

Back:
- Pelvis tilt (prone and supine)
- Back flexion (sit-ups)
- Back extension (push-ups)

NATA Competency Terms

Listed below is a list of musculoskeletal conditions/disorders that affect the head, neck, and/or spine. A valuable learning experience would be to define and review these conditions in a medical dictionary and/or sports medicine textbook.

Head/Face:

- Orbital Blowout Fracture
- Cauliflower Ear
- Conjunctivitis (pink eye)
- Corneal Abrasion
- Dental Cavities
- Detached Retina
- Deviated Septum
- Fractures
- Gingivitis
- Keratitis

- Otitis Externa
- Otitis Media
- Pericoronitis
- Peridontitis
- Periorbital Contusion (eyeball contusion)
- Skull Fracture
- Stye
- Temporomandibular Joint Dysfunction
- Tooth Abscess
- Tooth Extrusion

- Tooth Fracture
- Tooth Intrusion
- Tooth Luxation

Spinal Column:

- Nerve Root Compression
- Spinal Cord Injury
- Spondylitis
- Spondylosis
- Spondylolysis
- Spondylolisthesis

Review Questions - Chapter 10

Completion:

1. The seven _____ _____ make up the bones of the neck.

2. The brain is protected from trauma by the bones of the _____.

3. A _____ is defined as a shaking of the brain.

4. _____ is commonly referred to as a nosebleed.

5. When the brachial plexus becomes stretched or contused, a _____ _____ is produced.

6. Conjunctivitis is commonly referred to as _____ _____.

7. When evaluating a possible neck fracture _____ is not a factor.

8. The head weighs approximately _____ pounds.

9. An athlete with a head injury should be monitored at least _____ hours and carefully evaluated regularly for at least _____ week.

10. A concussion is defined as a _____ of the _____.

11. A person does not have to suffer a loss of _____ to have suffered a concussion.

12. Pressure on the brain will affect the _____ _____ system, causing various reactions of the body.

13. The first seven vertebrae are known as the _____ _____.

14. An injury to the neck could cause _____, or even _____.

15. A cervical neck injury involving a stretching the brachial plexus nerves is commonly called a _____ or _____.

Short Answer:

1. Name the three primary categories of intracranial hemorrhaging:

-
-
-

2. List three components of a comprehensive rehabilitation program:

-
-
-

3. Name two types of cervical rehabilitation:
-
-

4. Identify and define the three types of concussions.
-
-
-

5. Why should a football helmet not be removed from a player with a possible neck injury?

6. What are the symptoms of a cervical fracture or dislocation?

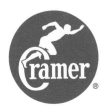

NOTES

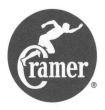

Chapter 11
The Shoulder and Upper Arm

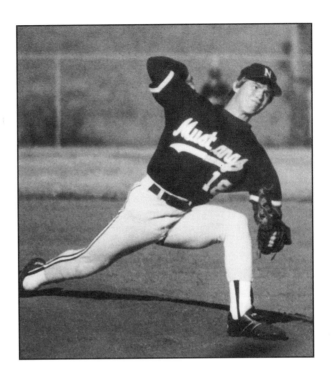

Educational Objectives

The learner should, at the completion of the chapter, be able to perform the following:

- Understand the anatomy of the shoulder complex and upper arm.
- Recognize the proper evaluation format for this region of the body.
- Identify the appropriate assessment tests for shoulder and upper arm injuries.
- Identify the common injuries associated with this region of the body.
- Understand the protocol for rehabilitation of the area.
- Recognize the proper taping and wrapping techniques for the shoulder and upper arm.
- Identify the NATA competencies for this region of the body.

The shoulder joint is the most mobile joint in the body. It can move up, down, forward, and backward; it allows the upper arm to assume an almost unlimited number of positions. Naturally, whatever position the shoulder and upper arm assume is yet another position in which they can become injured. The shoulder gains its mobility at the expense of stability. Many of its ligaments are loose, allowing greater movement of the bones.

This is a complex joint, which we will try to make more understandable. To help do this, discussion will center on two types of athletic injuries: those caused by direct trauma (contusions, sprains, dislocations, fractures, and strains) and those caused by indirect trauma.

Anatomy
Bones

The shoulder/upper arm complex is made up of three bones:

- Humerus, or upper arm bone
- Clavicle, or collar bone
- Scapula, or shoulder blade

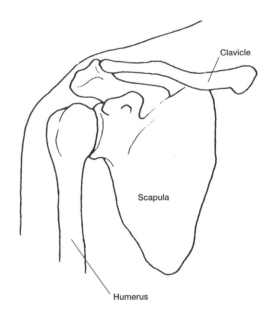

The Humerus

The humerus is the long bone of the upper arm. The skeletal articulation of the humerus and the scapula is structurally weak, but very mobile. This joint, the glenohumeral (GH) joint, is similar to the hip joint except that the socket is very shallow, allowing for greater movement.

The Clavicle

The clavicle supports the shoulder complex on the front of the body. There is no muscle or fat covering this bone, so it is easy to feel along its S-shaped length. Distally on the clavicle, you may be able to feel a projection. This is the point where the clavicle articulates with a part of the scapula known as the acromion process forming the acromioclavicular (AC) joint.

The clavicle also articulates with a second part of the scapula known as the coracoid process. These two bones are attached in both places by ligaments to form the coracoclavicular (CC) joint. The clavicle does not articulate with the humerus.

The Scapula

The scapula, which "floats" on the back of the rib cage, has two small, hooked projections. These projections, mentioned above, are the acromion process and the coracoid process. The scapula is held in place by the shoulder muscles.

Another section of the scapula is called the glenoid fossa, a shallow socket or cup on the lateral side of the scapula. This depression articulates with the spherical head of the humerus; the articulation is called the glenohumeral joint.

Ligaments

The primary ligaments of the shoulder complex allow for the tremendous mobility and movement associated with this region of the body. The strength and integrity of these structures, in conjunction with the muscles, account for the majority of the stability of the complex.

The following are considered the primary ligaments of the shoulder complex:
- **Costoclavicular**—limits clavicular movements.
- **Interclavicular**—strengthens the superior aspect of the joint capsule.
- **Acromioclavicular**—holds clavicle to acromion.
- **Coracoclavicular**—most important role in preventing separation of the clavicle from the scapula. Involved in impingement syndrome.

- **Coracohumeral**—strengthens the upper portion of the joint capsule.
- **Coracoacromial**—a ligament of the scapula from the coracoid process to acromion.

Muscles and Functions

Like the muscles of the knee, the muscles that cross the shoulder add a great deal of stability to the weak bony structure. The major muscles include the deltoid, which covers the top of the shoulder, and the pectoralis major, on the anterior aspect of the chest. These muscles attach to the shaft of the humerus.

Deeper muscles of the shoulder joint include a set of four muscles called the rotator cuff. These muscles surround the joint and are used mostly in throwing sports. For reference, their names are supraspinatus, infraspinatus, teres minor, and the subscapularis. Practically any exercise for back, chest and arm muscles will strengthen the shoulder.

The muscles of the shoulder complex assist with the stability, movement, and strength. The shoulder complex must be strong in order for the athlete to effectively participate in those sports that demand throwing as part of the game. The following muscles assist with the movement and strength of the shoulder complex:
- **Biceps**
- **Coracobrachialis**
- **Deltoid**
- **Infraspinatus**
- **Latissimus dorsi**
- **Levator scapulae**
- **Pectoralis major**
- **Pectoralis minor**
- **Rhomboids**
- **Serratus anterior**
- **Subscapularis**
- **Supraspinatus**
- **Teres major**
- **Teres minor**
- **Trapezius**
- **Triceps**

Joints

These three bones (humerus, clavicle, scapula) form four joints:

- Glenohumeral (GH)
- Acromioclavicular (AC)
- Sternoclavicular (SC)
- Coracoclavicular (CC)

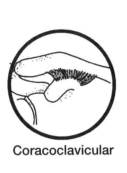 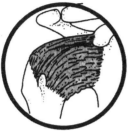

Coracoclavicular   Glenohumeral

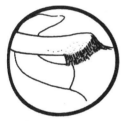 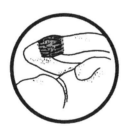

Sternoclavicular   Acromioclavicular

*The four Articulations of the shoulder (Source: **Essentials of Athletic Training, 3rd Ed., Daniel D. Arnheim, 1995.**)*

These joints are structurally unstable. In fact, attachment of the shoulder/upper arm complex to the skeletal system is made at one point only: the sternoclavicular (SC) joint. This attachment is the weak, but infrequently injured, articulation between the sternum and clavicle.

Range of Motion in Shoulder Joint

The range of motion of the shoulder joint is greater than any other major joint in the body. The shoulder complex allows for movement in all planes. The following are included in the range of motion for the shoulder complex.

- Flexion and Extension
- Abduction and Adduction
- Horizontal Abduction and Adduction
- Internal and External Rotation—with arm at the side of the body

- Internal and External Rotation—with the arm abducted to 90 degrees
- Circumduction

Range of Motion of Scapulothoracic

The following are included in the range of motion for the scapula (shoulder blades):

- Elevation
- Protraction
- Retraction
- Depression

Dermatomes

The sensation to the shoulder complex is provided by a number of nerves. The following nerves supply sensation to the skin and the shoulder complex:

- **C4**—which supplies the top of the shoulder
- **C5**—the lateral arm
- **C6**—the anterior and posterior arm
- **C7**—the posterior lateral arm
- **T1**—the medial arm
- **T2**—the axilla

Evaluation Format

The first purpose of an evaluation is to determine, to the best of your ability, if there is a fracture. Initially, a fracture should always be suspected. Signs of a fracture include, but are not limited to, direct or indirect pain, deformity, or a grating sound at the injury site. Some fractures are not accompanied by swelling or pain. If a fracture is suspected, the evaluation stops. The limb is splinted and the athlete is transported to proper medical authorities. Young athletes are especially susceptible to fractures; often, the ligaments are stronger than the bones. A force that will tear a ligament in a mature athlete will often avulse or pull away a chunk of bone, in the younger athlete.

The evaluation process to help determine the type of injury involves four steps: history, observation, palpation, and stress tests.

(H) History: This involves asking questions of the athlete to help determine the mechanism of injury.

111

Answers to these questions will help the physician in a diagnosis.

(O) Observation: Look for bleeding, deformity, swelling, discoloration and scars. The athletic trainer should compare the injured structure to the non-injured structure.

(P) Palpation: Any palpation (physical inspection) should take into account the emotional state of the athlete. Palpate the area away from the injury first, working towards the injury site. The entire area around the injury may be sore, but the athletic trainer should try to pinpoint the site of most severe pain. That will be the site where the most damage has been done. From knowledge of the shoulder's anatomy, the type and extent of injury can be evaluated. Involve the athlete in the evaluation as much as possible. Asking questions that require specific answers can provide valuable information.

(S) Stress Tests: With all tests, the athletic trainer is looking for pain and instability. Note: It is possible to further damage an injured shoulder through manipulation. Years of training are necessary before an athletic trainer would be considered competent to make stress tests and functional tests. These tests are well beyond the expertise of a student athletic trainer. **Functional Tests:** To determine if damage has been done to muscles, the athletic trainer uses functional tests, including range of motion. The athlete performs active and resistive exercises through all ranges of motion bilaterally against the athletic trainer's resistance. Pain or weakness could indicate muscle damage.

Refer to Chapter 2 for a full explanation of the H.O.P.S. injury evaluation format.

Assessment Tests

All injured joints should be properly evaluated. The purpose of a thorough evaluation is to enable the allied health professional to properly assess the severity of the injury and make recommendations regarding treatment and possible return to partici-

pation. Listed below is a review of evaluation techniques outlined in the *Sports Medicine Evaluation Series: Shoulder* published by Mosby Year Book, and sold by Cramer Products.

Glenohumeral Joint Stability Tests:
- Apprehension test
- Relocation test
- Anterior instability test
- Anterior/posterior translation test
- Posterior glenohumeral instability test
- Inferior drawer test or Feagin test

Rotator Cuff Impingement Tests:
- Rotator cuff impingement tests
- Full flexion test
- Flexion-internal rotation test

Rotator Cuff Muscular Strength Tests:
- Supraspinatus strength test (empty can test)
- Internal rotation strength test
- External rotation strength test

Internal Derangement Test:
- Glenoid labrum clunk test

Acromioclavicular Joint Tests:
- Acromioclavicular joint stability test
- Cross chest or horizontal adduction test

Sternoclavicular Joint Test:
- Sternoclavicular joint integrity test

Common Injuries
Conditions That Indicate an Athlete Should be Referred for Physician Evaluation:
- Suspected fracture, separation, or dislocation
- Gross deformity
- Significant loss of motion
- Significant or continued pain
- Joint instability
- Abnormal sensations that do not quickly go away, such as weakness or numbness
- Absent or weak pulse distal to the point of injury
- Any doubt regarding the severity or nature of the injury

Fractures

Fractures to the clavicle, humerus, and scapula (rare) can occur from a direct blow, or when an athlete falls on the shoulder or on an outstretched arm. In the latter case, the force is transmitted directly up the humerus. This can also be the mechanism of sprains to the various shoulder joints.

The clavicle is most often fractured in sports. The mechanism of injury is usually a direct blow, as the clavicle is relatively unprotected by muscles and ligaments. The majority of fractures occur in the middle third of the bone. The student athletic trainer may notice that the injured side appears a little lower than the uninjured side. First aid includes treating the athlete for shock, applying a sling and obtaining medical help.

Unlike the clavicle, the proximal end of the humerus is covered by a good deal of soft tissue. Therefore, with a fracture to the humerus in the shoulder area, the student athletic trainer may not notice the obvious deformity found with a fractured clavicle. A fractured humerus can result from a direct blow or from falling on an outstretched arm; a dislocation of the humeral head may also be accompanied by a fracture.

Fractures and dislocations of the head of the humerus should be treated as medical emergencies. This is because of the danger of tearing or impingement of the blood vessels and nerves that supply the arms. When pain, point tenderness, discoloration, and inability to move the arm point to a fracture of the humerus, the athlete should be treated for shock, have a sling applied, and taken to a medical facility.

Dislocations

The dislocation of the head of the humerus from its shallow joint is common in sports. Most often the injury is an anterior glenohumeral dislocation. All first-time dislocations should be considered to be fractures by the athletic trainer until X-ray reveals otherwise. Reduction of the dislocation should be handled by qualified medical personnel only. Damage to vessels and nerves can be a problem with this injury.

The anterior glenohumeral dislocation occurs when the arm is abducted and externally rotated, as sometimes occurs during arm tackling in football. Because of the displacement of the head of the humerus, the injured shoulder will look flat compared with the uninjured side. The athlete may hold the arm slightly abducted.

With this injury, supporting ligaments and muscles can be torn, causing hemorrhage. Immobilization of the arm in a comfortable position and application of cold packs are the first aid procedures. Shoulder dislocations require immobilization and a complete rehabilitation program to reduce the chance of recurrence.

Since most shoulder dislocations occur with the arm in abduction and externally rotated, rehabilitation should concentrate mainly on the movements of adduction and internal rotation. Athletes with chronic shoulder dislocations should be checked by the team physician because of the danger of arthritis development. Rehabilitation exercises should be assigned to strengthen strained muscles or those too weak for the activities of the sport.

Acromioclavicular (AC) Sprain

All the ligaments of the shoulder complex can be sprained, but the acromioclavicular sprain is the most common. The frequency of this injury is due to the location of the supporting ligaments on the tip of the shoulder. This injury is often referred to as a separated or knocked down shoulder.

The mechanism of injury is often a blow to the top of the shoulder or a fall on an outstretched arm. Depending on the force, the injury can be classified as first, second, or third degree.

The first degree sprain mildly stretches the acromioclavicular ligaments, resulting in pain between the clavicle and acromion process of the scapula. There is no deformity.

The second degree sprain has some tearing of the ligaments, resulting in clavicle displacement. The injured shoulder may appear to be knocked down. The athlete will not be able to move the arm very much without causing pain.

Third degree sprains result in extreme pain and obvious displacement of the clavicle. Surgery may be required.

A simple functional test that can be done to confirm an AC sprain is to have the athlete touch the opposite shoulder with the hand of the injured side. If there is an AC sprain, this movement may be painful, and perhaps even impossible to perform, depending on the severity of the injury.

First aid for AC sprains includes compression, cold, and stabilization of' the shoulder with a sling, the athlete should then be taken to a physician.

Flexibility and strengthening exercises should be undertaken for the entire shoulder area. Consult with the physician concerning when the exercises should be started and what kind of exercises should be done. If the physician allows the athlete to practice, the student athletic trainer can tape the shoulder to offer some protection. Modifications of this taping can be done for female athletes.

Contusions of the Shoulder

Both the muscles and the bones of the shoulder are often contused in sports. The point of' the clavicle is especially susceptible. After treatment, an athlete with a shoulder bruise might be able to continue to play if a foam rubber donut is used to take pressure off the point of tenderness. (The

Rehabilitation

Sending an athlete back to competition before healing is complete leaves the player susceptible to further injury. The best way to determine when healing is complete is by the absence of pain during stressful activity and by the return of full range of motion and strength.

Prior to the beginning of any rehabilitation exercise program, the athletic trainer should consult with a medical doctor to establish a program tailored for that individual athlete and the specific injury to be rehabilitated. The following exercises can be used as preventive or rehabilitative exercises:

Shoulder and Upper Arm:

- Non-gravity pendular movements
- Shoulder wheel
- Towel routine
- Swimming
- Light throwing

- Rowing
- Push-ups
- Military press
- T-Bar exercises
- Arm pulley

- Band Exercises

The goal of injury rehabilitation is to return the injured athlete to competition as quickly as possible, but not so quickly as to aggravate the existing injury. Components of a rehabilitation protocol would include:

- Range-of-motion exercises
- Resistance exercises

- Sport specific exercises

Exercises

Exercises for the shoulder complex injury would include passive and active exercises. Those exercises that require the athletic trainer to assist the injured athlete are considered passive and are typically done early in the rehabilitation process. Those exercises that the athlete is able to perform on their own are active exercises and follow the advanced stages of the rehabilitation protocol. Exercises, whether passive or active, should not make the injury worse, although there may be pain and discomfort associated with the exercise.

mechanism and implications of this injury are similar to the thigh contusion; see Chapter 7.)

We have already discussed some of the numerous muscles that help give the shoulder joint its mobility. These muscles all have the potential of being strained. If an athlete reports to you with shoulder pain and gives no history of falling on the joint or being hit, suspect a muscle strain.

When palpating the area, the student athletic trainer may note soreness or pain primarily in the soft tissue. Manual resistance to every movement the shoulder can make may help reveal the injured muscle. As the student athletic trainer resists the athlete's flexion, extension and other movements, one particular range of motion may produce the most pain. After identifying the strain, the student athletic trainer can pack the area with cold packs.

The shoulder, if immobilized, is more likely to lose its flexibility and motion than any other joint. It is therefore necessary for the athlete to regain full range-of-motion as quickly as possible.

Common causes of shoulder muscle strains are lack of strength, overuse, improper technique and inadequate warm-up. In addition to the muscles, other soft tissue structures in the shoulder can be injured by the repetitive actions and forces of sports.

Several bursae separate the deltoid and rotator cuff muscles and also cushion the muscles around the AC joint. These bursae are also susceptible to injury. Despite a relatively poor blood supply in this area, minor muscle strains and irritation of the bursae heal rapidly. Overuse by the athlete, however, can further strain the muscles and compound the minor tissue damage. These conditions of overuse are called tendinitis (if the problem is muscular) and bursitis (if the damage is to the bursae). If left untreated, swelling can cause subtle changes in motion that could damage the deep rotator cuff muscles.

Preventive/Supportive Techniques

Taping is a time-honored and time-consuming tradition. It is also a very expensive practice. Whether to tape healthy body parts is a decision the athletic trainer will have to make.

All injured joints should be taped initially. The purpose of taping is to keep the joint from moving so the ligaments won't be stretched further. Listed below is a review of techniques that are outlined in *The Comprehensive Manual of Taping and Wrapping Techniques* published by Cramer Products.

Shoulder and Upper Arm:
• Acromioclavicular joint taping
• Glenohumeral joint taping

NATA Competency Terms

Listed below is a list of musculoskeletal conditions/disorders that affect the shoulder girdle. A valuable learning experience would be to define and review these conditions in a medical dictionary and/or sports medicine textbook.

• Blocker's exostosis	• Fracture	• Strain
• Bursitis	• Nerve injury	• Tenosynovitis
• Contusion	• Rotator cuff strain	
• Dislocation/subluxation	• Sprain	

Chapter 11 - Review Questions

Completion:

1. The _____ _____ is the point where the clavicle articulates with the scapula.

2. The clavicle does not articulate with the _____.

3. If a fracture is suspected the evaluation _____.

4. Palpate the area _____ from the injury first, working _____ the injury site.

5. A relocation test, tests the stability of the _____ _____.

6. The _____ is the most often fractured bone in sports.

7. A _____ _____ is the most common shoulder dislocation.

8. _____ _____ _____ is an example of shoulder and upper arm taping.

9. The three bones that make up the shoulder/upper arm complex are the _____, the _____, and the _____. These bones form how many joints _____?

10. Where does the shoulder/upper arm complex attach to the skeletal system _____?

11. The shoulder gains mobility at the expense of _____.

12. The _____ end of the clavicle articulates with the sternum. The _____ end articulates with the acromion process.

13. _____ attach the scapula to the clavicle.

14. Resistance to shoulder movements can often reveal an injury to a specific _____.

15. Shoulder dislocation should always be evaluated by a _____.

16. With a shoulder dislocation, you should always suspect a _____.

17. First aid treatment for an AC sprain includes _____, _____ and _____.

18. Contusions of the distal end of the clavicle are called _____ _____.

19. The four deep muscles that stabilize the head of the humerus into the glenoid fossa are referred to as the _____ _____.

Short Answer:

1. Name three components of a rehabilitation protocol:

-
-
-

2. Name two shoulder rehabilitative exercises:

-
-

3. Name two shoulder NATA competency terms:

-
-

4. Name 6 muscles that add stability to the shoulder?

-
-
-
-
-
-

5. Define strain:

6. Name an internal derangement test.

7. What is the purpose of taping?

8. What is the rotator cuff?

9. Describe first aid for a fractured clavicle.

10. Define and describe the SC and AC joints.

11. What is a common mechanism of shoulder sprains?

12. Why is a fracture of the clavicle usually more noticeable than a fracture of the proximal head of the humerus?

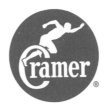

NOTES

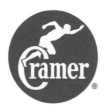

Chapter 12

The Elbow, Forearm, Wrist, and Hand

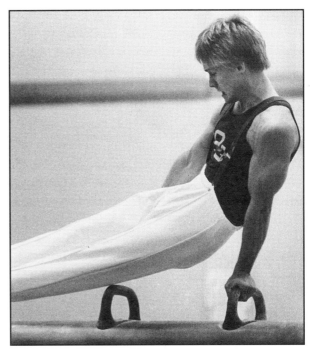

Educational Objectives

The learner should, at the completion of the chapter, be able to perform the following:

- Understand the anatomy of the elbow, forearm, wrist, and hand.
- Recognize the appropriate evaluation format for this region of the body.
- Identify the common injuries to the elbow, fore arm, wrist, and hand.
- Understand the protocol for rehabilitation exercises for this area of the body.
- Recognize the proper taping and wrapping techniques for the elbow, forearm, wrist, and hand.
- Identify the NATA competencies for this region of the body.

The elbow joint is an intricate collection of bones, muscles, ligaments and nerves. It permits the movements of flexion, extension, pronation and supination. Many sports place specific demands on the elbow, and each movement can lead to a specific injury. The elbow joint often delivers, and sometimes receives, accidental blows that can cause bruising, fracture, dislocation or nerve damage. Massive stresses are placed on the elbow in throwing sports. Racquet sports bring their own special demands to the elbow joint. In fact, the elbow is the most frequently injured joint in tennis, a tennis player uses the elbow to both propel and twist the racquet.

Anatomy - Elbow

The elbow joint is composed of three bones:
- **Humerus**
- **Radius**
- **Ulna**

The humerus, the largest bone of the arm, has two articulating condyles at its distal end. Of the two bones of the lower arm, the ulna acts as a stationary axle; the radius turns around it as the forearm and hand rotate. Hang your arm at your side with the palm facing forward. The small bony prominence closest to the body is the medial epicondyle of the humerus. The lateral epicondyle is on the opposite side. Ligaments and tendons use the distal knobs of the humerus as a base of attachment.

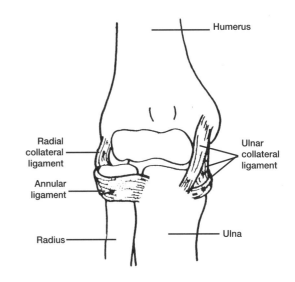

The Elbow

121

The medial condyle articulates with the ulna of the lower arm to allow flexion and extension of the elbow. The lateral condyle of the humerus articulates with the radius, allowing pronation and supination of the lower arm and hand. The elbow joint is considered to have very strong ligamentous and muscular support. The elbow joint is stabilized by medial and lateral collateral ligaments. The medial collateral ligament is attached to the humerus and the ulna; the lateral collateral ligament is attached to the humerus and the radius. Adding further to the elbow's stability is the annular ligament. This ligament attaches to the ulna and completely encircles the head of the radius. The annular ligament helps keep the radius and ulna from separating.

The muscles that control the elbow's movement originate above the elbow, on the humerus and the scapula (shoulder blade). These muscles include:

• **Biceps** originates on the humerus and scapula, splits into two parts, and attach individually to the ulna and radius. The primary function of the biceps group is flexion of the elbow.

• **Triceps** originate at three sites and attaches to the ulna. This muscle group's primary function is extension of the elbow.

• **Brachialis** originate low on the humerus, attaching to the ulna. The brachialis group also assists in elbow flexion.

The numerous muscles that control the movements of the forearm, wrist, and fingers originate on the two epicondyles of the humerus. Muscles that allow the forearm to flex and pronate are the flexor capri radialis, flexor capri ulnaris, flexor digitorum sublimis, and flexor pollicis longus. Forearm muscles that permit extension and supination are the extensor digitorum communis, extensor capri radialis brevis, extensor capri ulnaris, and extensor pollicis longus.

The elbow is made up of two joints, called the humeroulnar and humeroradial. Within these joints, the three ligaments that support this joint are the ulnar collateral, annular, and the radial collateral. Range of motion in the elbow joint is:

• Flexion—135 degrees plus

• Extension—0 /-5 degrees
• Supination—90 degrees
• Pronation—90 degrees

Anatomy - Wrist and Hand

Wrist and Hand - Bones

The wrist and hand is made up of twenty seven bones. They are:
• Navicular
• Lunate
• Triquetrum
• Pisiform
• Trapezium
• Trapezoid
• Capitate
• Hamate
• Metacarpals (5)
• Phalanges (14)

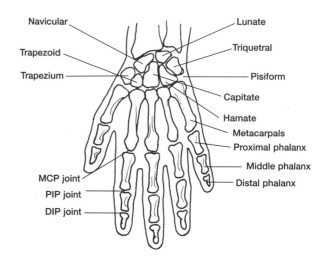

Bones of the hand and wrist

Wrist and Hand - Muscles
• Flexor/Extensor carpi radialis
• Flexor/Extensor carpi ulnaris
• Flexor/Extensor pollicis longis
• Flexor/Extensor pollicis brevis

- Flexor/Extensor digiti
- Abductor/Adductor pollicis
- Interossei palmares
- Opponens pollicis
- Opponens digiti minimi

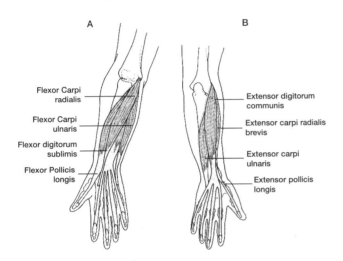

*Muscles of the Hand and Wrist (Source: **Essentials of Athletic Training, 3rd Ed., Arnheim, 1993**.)*

Within the wrist and hand, there are numerous joints that allow movement. Here is a brief listing of these joints: radiocarpal, midcarpal, carpometacarpal, intercarpal, metacarpophalangeal, and interphalangeal (which include DIP and PIP joints in the fingers). The muscles surrounding the wrist and hand include abductor pollicis brevis, flexor pollicis brevis, opponens pollicis, adductor pollicis, abductor digiti minimi, flexor digiti minimi brevis, opponens digiti minimi, palmar interossei, and dorsal interossei.

Basic range of motion to the **wrist and hand** would include these movements:

- Flexion
- Extension
- Radial Deviation
- Ulnar Deviation

Basic range of motion to the fingers would include:

- Flexion and extension at metacarpophalangeal joints
- Flexion and extension at I.P. joints

- Abduction and adduction at the metacarpophalangeal joints
- Thumb flexion and extension at the M.C.P. and I.P. joint
- Thumb abduction and adduction at the carpometacarpal joint
- Opposition

Dermatomes of the Elbow, Wrist and Hand are:

- C5—Supplies the lateral aspect of the upper arm.
- C6—supplies sensation to the thumb, index, and half of the middle finger.
- C7—supplies the middle finger with contributions from C6 & C8.
- C8—supplies the ring and little finger.
- T1—supplies the medial upper arm and axilla.

Evaluation Format

The first purpose of an evaluation is to determine, to the best of your ability, if there is a fracture. Initially, a fracture should always be suspected. Signs of a fracture include, but are not limited to, direct or indirect pain, deformity, or a grating sound at the injury site. Some fractures are not accompanied by swelling or pain. If a fracture is suspected, the evaluation stops. The limb is splinted and the athlete is transported to proper medical authorities. Young athletes are especially susceptible to fractures; often, the ligaments are stronger than the bones. A force that will tear a ligament in a mature athlete will often avulse, or pull away a chunk of bone, in the younger athlete.

The evaluation process to help determine the type of injury involves four steps: history, observation, palpation, and stress tests.

(H) History: This involves asking questions of the athlete to help determine the mechanism of injury. Answers to these questions will help the physician in a diagnosis.

(O) Observation: Look for bleeding, deformity, swelling, discoloration, and scars. The athletic trainer should compare the injured area to the non-injured area.

(P) Palpation: Any palpation (physical inspection) should take into account the emotional state of the athlete. Palpate the area away from the injury first, working toward the injury site. The entire area around the injury may be sore, but the athletic trainer should try to pinpoint the site of most severe pain. That will be the site where the most damage has been done. From knowledge of the elbow, forearm and wrist's anatomy, the type and extent of injury can be evaluated. Involve the athlete in the evaluation as much as possible. Asking questions that require specific answers can provide valuable information.

(S) Stress Tests: With all tests, the athletic trainer is looking for pain and instability. Note: It is possible to further damage an injured elbow, forearm or wrist joint through manipulation. Years of training are necessary before an athletic trainer would be considered competent to make stress tests and functional tests. These tests are well beyond the expertise of a student athletic trainer. Functional Tests: To determine if damage has been done to muscles, the athletic trainer uses functional tests, including range of motion. The athlete performs active and resistive exercises through all ranges of motion bilaterally against the athletic trainer's resistance. Pain or weakness could indicate muscle damage.

Refer to Chapter 2 for a full explanation of the H.O.P.S. injury evaluation format.

Assessment Tests

All injured joints should be properly evaluated. The purpose of a thorough evaluation is to enable the allied health professional to properly assess the severity of the injury and make recommendations regarding treatment and possible return to participation.

Elbow

Tests for Ligament Stability:
- Valgus or abduction stress test (full extension and 20 degrees flexion)
- Varus or adduction stress test (full extension and 20 degrees flexion)

Epicondylitis Tests—Lateral:
- Resisted wrist extension test
- Resisted long finger extension test
- Palmar flexion-pronation stretch test

Epicondylitis Tests—Medial:
- Resisted wrist flexion test
- Wrist extension-supination stretch test

Neurological Dysfunction Tests:
- Tinel sign test
- The pronator teres syndrome test
- Pinch grip test

Wrist and Hand

Bony Integrity Tests:
- Anatomical snuffbox compression test
- Murphy's sign

Ligamentous Tests (fingers/thumb):
- PIP and DIP collateral ligament test
- MCP collateral ligament test
- Gamekeeper's thumb test

Musculoskeletal Tests:
- Finkelstein's test
- Flexor digitorum superficialis test
- Flexor digitorum profundus test
- Mallet finger test
- Boutonniere deformity test

Carpal Tunnel Tests:
- Phalen's test or wrist press test
- Tinel's sign at the wrist

Common Injuries - Elbow

Conditions That Indicate an Athlete Should be Referred for Physician Evaluation
- Gross deformity about the elbow or forearm
- Suspected fracture or dislocation
- Significant swelling and pain
- Joint instability
- Loss of sensation (motor or sensory)
- Loss of motion

Bursitis (Olecranon)—inflammation of the bursa causing the area to feel thick. Results from a blow to the tip of the elbow if traumatic, or may be a chronic inflammatory process.

Contusion—a bruising of tissue usually on the ulnar side of the forearm.

Dislocation/Subluxation—most common is the posterior displacement of the ulna and radius in relationship to the humerus. Usually occurs because of a fall on an outstretched hand with the elbow in extension. Dislocations that remain displaced appear deformed with the olecranon process prominent and the athlete expressing pain. May have an associated fracture.

Epicondylitis—inflammation of the epicondyle and the tissues adjoining the epicondyle to the humerus (pitcher's elbow—medial epicondyle, tennis elbow—lateral epicondyle).

Forearm Splints—repeated static contractions resulting in a strain of the forearm muscles (cheerleaders).

Sprain—uncommon in the elbow joint because this is a relatively stable joint. Injuries involving the ligamentous system most commonly result from partial dislocation or subluxation. More common to the ulnar collateral ligament complex.

Common Injuries - Wrist and Hand

Barton Fracture—fracture of the distal end of the radius into the wrist joint.

Bennett Fracture—fracture of the proximal end or base of the first metacarpal, often associated with subluxation of the carpometacarpal joint.

Boutonniere Deformity—results from an injury to the central slip of the extensor tendon; the proximal interphalangeal joint is flexed and the distal interphalangeal and metacarpophalangeal joints are in a hyperextended position.

Carpal Tunnel Syndrome—symptoms resulting from constriction in the carpal tunnel and pressure on the median nerve.

Colles' Fracture—fracture of the distal end of the radius in which the fragment is displaced dorsally.

Ganglion—herniated tendon.

Navicular Fracture—the carpal most often fractured; results from a fall on extended wrist, often leads to non-union of the bone fragments due to its poor blood supply. Usually severe pain is located in the anatomical snuffbox.

Subungual Hematoma—accumulation of blood under the fingernail.

Rehabilitation

Prior to initiating a rehabilitative program, a proper evaluation must be completed. All injuries should be thoroughly evaluated by a physician or athletic trainer with recommendations concerning proper treatment and rehabilitative exercises outlined. Listed below are types of exercises for each joint.

Wrist and Hand:
- Wrist flexion
- Wrist extension
- Wrist ulnar deviation
- Wrist radial deviation
- Finger flexion
- Finger extension
- Finger/thumb extension
- Hand squeeze
- Finger abduction
- Pinch grip
- Hand squeeze
- Lateral/key pinch grip

Elbow:
- Elbow flexion
- Elbow extension
- Pronation
- Supination

Preventive/Supportive Techniques

Listed below is review of the taping and wrapping techniques outlined in the textbook titled *The Comprehensive Manual of Taping and Wrapping Techniques* published by Cramer Products. Please review this text for a complete description on how to apply these preventive/supportive techniques.

Elbow
- Elbow hyperextension
- Elbow epicondylitis wrap
- Forearm splint taping

Wrist and Hand
- Wrist taping
- Thumb spica taping
- Thumb c-lock taping
- Finger splint taping
- Collateral interphalangeal joint taping
- Hyperextension of phalanges taping
- Contusion of hand

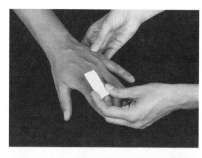
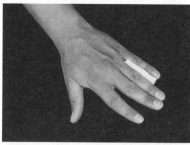
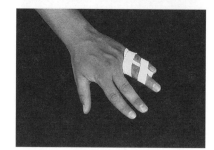

One of the best ways to protect a sprained finger is with "buddy" taping, in which the injured finger is taped to the stronger adjacent finger for support.

NATA Competency Terms

Listed below is a list of musculoskeletal conditions/disorders that affect the elbow, wrist and /or hand. A valuable learning experience would be to define and review these conditions in a medical dictionary and/or sports medicine textbook.

Elbow:
- Bursitis
- Epiphyseal plate injury
- Epicondylitis
- Fracture
- Nerve injury
- Osteochondritis dissecans
- Supracondylar fracture
- Ulnar nerve contusion
- Volkman's fracture (ischemia)

Wrist And Hand:
- Baseball finger
- Boxers fracture
- Dislocation
- Epiphyseal plate injury
- Felon
- Fracture
- Paronychia
- Smith's fracture
- Sprain

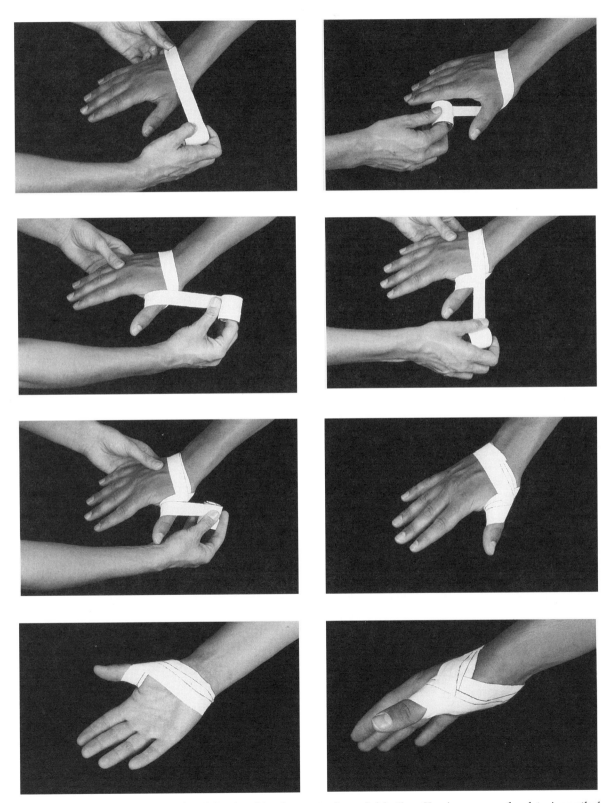

Taping the thumb can help prevent it from being forced into hyperextension and abduction. Here is a common thumb taping method.

Chapter 12 - Review Questions

Completion:

1. _____ signs are always suspected first in an evaluation of the elbow, wrist, hand, and forearm.

2. Just as in the knee, _____ and _____ tests assess the elbow collateral ligaments.

3. The anatomical snuff box test can help identify a possible _____ of the _____ bone.

4. Pitcher elbow is a problem of the _____ _____.

5. _____ is the accumulation of blood under the fingernail.

6. Pronation and supination are suggested exercises for _____ rehabilitation.

7. The bones that form the elbow are the _____, _____ and _____.

8. The three wrist bones most often fractured are the _____, _____ and the _____.

9. The _____ is similar to the femur of the leg, as both have two _____ at their _____ or lower ends.

10. Of the two bones of the lower arm, the _____ acts as a stationary axle.

11. The lateral condyle of the humerus articulates with the radius, allowing _____ and _____ of the lower arm and hand.

12. The elbow joint has very _____ ligamentous and muscular support. As is the knee, the elbow joint is stabilized by medial and lateral _____ ligaments.

13. Helping to stabilize the elbow joint, by attaching to the ulna and encircling the head of the radius, is the _____ ligament.

14. The three muscle groups that control the movement of the elbow are the _____, _____, and the _____.

15. Tennis elbow is often an inflammation of the _____ _____.

16. The wrist joint is formed by the distal ends of the _____ and _____, and by the eight _____ bones.

Short Answer:

1. Name the four ligaments of the elbow joint.

-
-
-
-

2. List two suggested exercises for rehabilitation of the wrist and hand.

-
-

3. Name the eight bones that make up the wrist.

-
-
-
-
-
-
-
-

4. Name the three groups of bones of the hand.

-
-
-

5. List two supportive techniques for the wrist and hand.

-
-

6. What might happen if a navicular fracture is mistaken for a severe sprain?

7. What is the evaluation process used in this text?

8. Why are elbow dislocations potentially serious?

NOTES

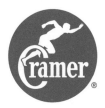

Chapter 13
Special Considerations In Athletic Training

Educational Objectives

The learner should, at the completion of the chapter, be able to perform the following:

- Recognize the various environmental conditions that affect sport.
- Recognize the signs and symptoms of nutritional/eating disorders among athletes.
- Identify the various skin conditions that are common in athletic training situations.
- Understand the difference between bacterial and viral infections.
- Understand the legal and ethical issues that face athletic trainers.
- Identify the common medical illnesses that are seen in athletic training.

Environmental Conditions

There are three basic environmental conditions that impact athletic performance: heat, cold, and altitude. All three can have a negative effect on performance. To counter this the athletic trainer, coach, and athlete must prepare for these conditions. The guidelines for prevention and symptoms of environmental distress are discussed in the following paragraphs.

Heat Related Conditions

High temperatures and elevated humidity can negatively impact athletic performance, adversely affect health and even threaten life. While environmental heat problems most often strike football players, all athletes are susceptible.

Exercise generates heat, which the body must dissipate. If too much heat is retained by the body, cells will literally cook, and the victim can die. The

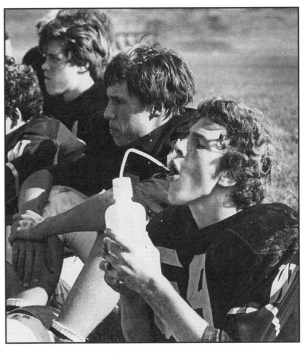

body cools itself mainly through the sweating mechanism; heat is carried away from the body as perspiration evaporates. This cooling process can be interrupted in two ways: the humidity can be so high that sweat does not evaporate, or the thermoregulatory system of the athlete can be disrupted, causing sweating to cease.

The coach and student athletic trainer can help prevent heat related problems in several ways:

1) Prehydration and rehydration: Heavy fluid intake before, during, and after practice will help insure that athletes function efficiently and safely. The weight an athlete loses through exertion is almost entirely fluid loss. A fluid loss of as little as 3% of total body weight can adversely affect endurance and coordination; it can also start the athlete down the road to heat illness.

There are several reasons for athletes to prehydrate. First, they need to replace lost fluid from the previous practice session. Second, thirst is not an accurate indicator of the need for fluid. A thirsty person will feel rehydrated well before the adequate intake of fluids. Third, drinking too much water at one time will give the athlete an uncomfortable feeling; several smaller doses of water are better than one large amount.

One strategy for replacing fluids is to drink cold water using the following formula:
- 34 oz. two hours before practice
- 13 - 17 oz. 15 minutes before practice
- 13 - 17 oz. every 30 minutes during practice

During peak exertion, when gastric emptying is most crucial, it is better to give your athletes plain water. Another option is to serve them electrolyte drinks diluted even more than package directions indicate, which will replace lost electrolytes without significantly slowing gastric emptying time. It is best to use electrolyte drinks before and after practice, when gastric emptying time is less crucial. **DO NOT DENY AN ATHLETE WATER OR REST AT ANY TIME.**

2) Acclimatization: While humans can not get used to being deprived of water, they can get better acclimated to hot weather. This process can take 1-2 weeks of working out in heat with gradually increased intensity.

3) Wear proper clothing: Light, loose fitting clothing will allow air to move over the body. Heat can be trapped by clothing that binds. Helmets should be taken off during breaks. Do not allow athletes to work out in rubberized clothing or sweatsuits in the false belief that they are accelerating weight loss. (The weight loss will be easily replaced fluid, not fat loss.) Perspiration will be trapped, the cooling process will be interrupted, and the stage will be set for dehydration and heat illness.

4) Use weight charts: The student athletic trainer can weigh all players before and after each practice. Athletes who do not regain their lost water weight by the start of the next practice should be encouraged to replace fluids. If there is significant fluid loss, the team physician should be contacted.

5) Do not give salt tablets: The amount of water needed to balance the salt intake is much more than the athlete can comfortably drink; the best method for increasing salt is during meals. Fluids are much

more important than salt in avoiding heat problems.

6) Be prepared to give first aid: Know the signs of heat exhaustion and heat stroke and be prepared to provide first aid.

Heat Stroke

Heat stroke is caused by high body temperature, dehydration and salt loss. The body's mechanisms for dissipating heat will have stopped working, and a tremendous increase in body temperature will occur rapidly. Heat stroke is a medical emergency and must be treated as a life-threatening situation. The signs and symptoms of heat stroke are:
- The victim may be dizzy, weak, mentally confused, or have a sense of doom.
- The victim's skin may be extremely dry and will appear flushed. The pulse will be strong and rapid.
- The victim's temperature will be very high, the skin will feel hot to the touch. Rectally, the temperature will be above 105 degrees, and it may range as high as 109 degrees.
- With little warning, the victim may become unconscious .

First Aid Procedures: Coaches and athletic trainers must review first aid treatment with the team physician before the season starts. Because heat stroke is caused by the body's acute inability to lose heat rapidly, the following steps must be taken immediately:
- Make immediate arrangements to have the athlete transported to the nearest medical facility. Severe neurological, circulatory, and hepatic (liver) conditions may occur if quick and definitive medical attention is not sought.
- Remove all clothing and pads and place the athlete in the coolest available place.
- Cool the athlete's body by any means possible. Some experts recommend placing the victim in an ice bath; others fear this could cause too great a shock to the victim's system. Any method that helps lower the body temperature, cold water,

chemical cooling packs, ice rubbed vigorously over the body, should be used.
- If the patient is conscious and can cooperate, give cold drinks to aid in heat loss.

Heat Exhaustion

Heat exhaustion may be difficult to recognize. Its symptoms generally are less severe than those of heat stroke and vital signs may even appear normal. Coaches and athletic trainers should look for the following signs to determine if the victim is suffering from heat exhaustion:
- The victim may experience progressive weakness and incoordination.
- The skin is usually moist and clammy, and may be pale or gray.
- The pulse may be weak and slightly more rapid than normal (less than 100 beats per minute).
- The pupils may be dilated.
- The victim is usually conscious, but fainting may occur.
- The victim may be suffering from muscle cramps.

First Aid Procedures: Heat exhaustion is an emergency situation, but it usually is not life-threatening. First aid for heat exhaustion includes:
- The athlete should lie in a cool place out of the sun.
- Encourage the athlete to drink as much cool water as possible.

- Remove excess clothing and rub the athlete's body with a cool, wet cloth.
- The athlete should be instructed to stay out of the heat until seen by a physician. Take the athlete to a hospital in case of other complications.

It is essential that coaches, staff athletic trainers and student athletic trainers know the signs of heat exhaustion and heat stroke. Remember that heat problems can strike athletes in any sport.

The following chart should help the athletic trainer determine whether the athlete is experiencing heat stroke or heat exhaustion.

Cold Weather Precautions
Fluid Replacement

Dehydration, the primary cause of heat illness, can occur not only in hot, humid weather, but also during the coldest days of the year. Athletes can lose 5 to 10 pounds of fluid weight during one hot weather practice session; strenuous winter workouts in the gym can have the same effect. In addition, during the winter the body loses essential fluids in ways besides sweating. The air inside heated buildings and outdoors is almost always drier during the winter than in the summer. It must be warmed and moisturized before it can be absorbed by the lungs. During this process, the body uses fluids and energy at a very rapid rate, calling for continuous fluid replacement.

Signs and Symptoms

Signs	Heat Exhaustion	Heat Stroke
Face	Pale	Red and Flushed
Skin	Moist	Hot and Dry
Temperature	Normal (98.6)	Extremely High (104+)
Pulse	Weak/Rapid	Strong/Rapid
Level of Consciousness	Usually Conscious	Usually Unconscious

Note: *The non-white athlete will still exhibit a paling of the skin, but you need to examine the inner lip and gum area. The same holds true for red and flushed skin. Look at the lip and gum area to see a discoloration of the non-white athlete.*

The body's thirst mechanism isn't always accurate, especially in the winter. Athletes may not feel as thirsty as they did on that hot August afternoon, but they may be just as much in need of fluid replacement.

Frostbite

In severely cold conditions, frostbite becomes another major concern for athletes. Late-autumn football games are sometimes played in sub-freezing air temperatures. When combined with wind, these low temperatures can freeze unprotected skin tissue. The most susceptible areas are the fingers, toes, ears and exposed parts of the face. Common frostbite warning signals include a tingling or burning sensation, pain, numbness, and discoloration of the skin (frostbitten areas have a yellow-white, waxy appearance). In extreme cold, however, flesh may freeze quickly, without warning, due to the cold's anesthetizing effect on the skin.

Keeping cold and dampness away from the skin is the best protection against frostbite. You can also help ward off frostbite with physical actions, such as wiggling fingers and toes, making faces, and working the muscles to increase the supply of blood to various areas. If frostbite should occur, treatment depends on the extent of damage. Be sure to notify your athletic trainer if you suspect that an athlete is suffering from frostbite.

Hypothermia

Any athlete who participates in outdoor recreation should guard against excessive heat loss and recognize the following progressive signs of hypothermia, a potentially fatal condition. Those signs include:

- Constant shivering; this is an attempt by the body to generate heat.
- Apathy, slurring of speech, listlessness, involuntary muscle movement, croaky voice, sleepiness, and generalized rigidity of muscles.
- Unconsciousness, pupils that are abnormally dilated and that react sluggishly to light, and very slow pulse and respiratory rates.
- Freezing of hands and/or feet.

If nothing is done to prevent further loss of body heat or to start the warming process once these stages have begun, heartbeat and respiration can fail as quickly as an hour and a half after shivering starts, leading swiftly to death. For this reason, prompt initial care is of utmost importance. If you suspect that an athlete is suffering from hypothermia, take him to a warm area, remove any wet clothing and gradually warm the body in warm, dry blankets. Immediately notify emergency personnel, as well as your athletic trainer.

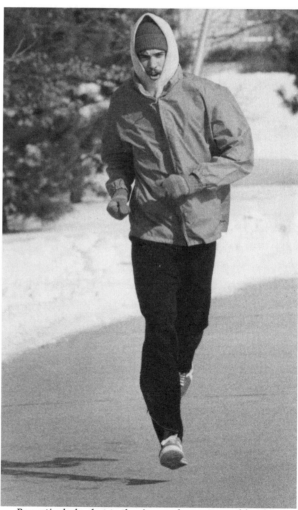

Be particularly alert to the signs and symptoms of frostbite and hypothermia during cold-weather workouts.

Altitude

The third type of environmental condition that can be experienced by athletes is altitude. When an athlete trains at one altitude level and then must compete at another altitude level, these athletes can experience an impact on their performances.

Typically the negative impact occurs when an athlete who has trained at a low altitude level must compete at a significantly higher altitude level. This impacts performance because the higher altitude has less oxygen concentration. This makes it more difficult for the athlete to supply the required amount of oxygen to the body's systems.

This negative impact is usually seen with sports that are aerobic in nature. Anaerobic sporting events result in less of an impact because the event is over before the body experiences an oxygen debt.

To avoid this condition, athletes should be given the opportunity to train at the higher elevations for a period of time that allows their bodies to adjust to the rarefied oxygen atmosphere.

Other Environmental Conditions

One additional condition that can impact athletes is circadian dysrythymia. This is when the body's internal clock is confused. This occurs when athletes travel across numerous time zones and is typically seen when the athlete travels from the west to the east. Both the eating and sleeping rhythm are disrupted and the athlete's internal clock is trying to adjust, but is having difficulty because of the day/night sequence.

Nutrition and Eating Disorders

What and when an athlete eats can affect performance. Common advice is that an individual should wait an hour or more after eating to exercise. Although athletes with full stomachs will not necessarily have performance problems, there is some truth in this advice. It is a fact that when there is food in the stomach, more blood is required for digestion, and that during physical activity, more blood is needed by the moving muscles. Therefore, unless an adequate amount of blood can be pumped out in order to fulfill both needs, either the digestion process or the working muscles will be in short supply of blood. This can cause stomach cramping, digestive upsets, and overall muscle weakness.

Athletes vary in their ability to exercise after eating (or without eating). Some complain of becoming dizzy or weak during practice unless they have a snack beforehand. This can be prevented by eating a substantial, well-balanced lunch. Normal gastric emptying (from the stomach into the small intestine) can take from one to four hours, depending on the composition of the meal. High carbohydrate and liquid meals will pass through the digestive system more quickly than meals high in fats and solids.

Another factor in digestion rate is how well food is chewed. The stomach has to work harder on food that hasn't been adequately chewed, and it holds it for a longer period of time. This often causes a feeling of fullness or bloating.

If an athlete eats a good lunch and still experiences hunger pangs or weakness during and after practice, they may need an extra snack, as long as the feeling of having food in the stomach does not interfere with their athletic performance. However, they should select small portions of foods that are not spicy or bulky and that are easily digested. Pre-activity foods should exclude the following items:

- Fatty foods. These are digested slowly and can interfere with efficiency in exercise.
- Gas forming foods that can cause discomfort and detract from physical abilities.
- Salt tablets; the average diet already contains enough salt.
- Special "magic" foods.
- Nutritional supplements are useless, costly, and potentially dangerous.

A wise selection for pre- and post-activity eating is a menu that is low in fat content, non-gaseous, nonalcoholic, well-balanced, high in carbohydrates, and high in fiber. A good example would be a meal that includes broiled chicken, a baked potato, green beans, skim milk, and a baked apple. To replace diminished glycogen stores, post-exercise menus should also emphasize carbohydrate-rich foods. Fluid replacement should include two cups of liquid for every pound lost. Suggest to athletes that they avoid consuming beverages containing caffeine, such as soft drinks, tea, and coffee, before practices and games. Beverages containing caffeine stimulate the flow of urine, which may cause discomfort during competition or decrease the body's water level before competition, adversely affecting performance. Instead, athletes should drink plenty of plain water or electrolyte drinks to insure that they are well hydrated before practices and games.

Remember that the total diet consumed during the days before the event is far more important than the meal eaten immediately prior to strenuous exercise.

Anorexia Nervosa

This is one of the two eating disorders most commonly associated with athletics. This disorder is characterized by a person refusing to eat or not eating enough to maintain normal body functions. This is commonly seen in the sports that have a high body image profile. Although the disorder can occur with any athlete, the sports most affected include, but are not limited to, cheerleaders, gymnastics, cross country, wrestling, figure skating, and those sports that have weight classifications or weight limitations.

Bulimia

This is the second of the two eating disorders commonly associated with participation in sports. This particular disorder is characterized by overeating (binge) and then vomiting (purge). The athlete will consume large quantities of food and immediately vomit the food. This routine by the athlete is an attempt to gain essential energy requirements, but not the weight associated with the food. This psychological problem is best handled by a person qualified in psychological disorders. The best plan of action by the athletic trainer is to refer the athlete to the most qualified health care provider.

Food and Vitamin Supplements

While food is important for both general health and athletic performance, the nutritional needs of athletes are no different from those of their non-

athletic peers. Misinformation concerning the role of nutrition and athletics can be confusing to the coach and athlete, sometimes leading to the improper and unnecessary use of food and vitamin supplements. There are no "super foods" or wonder diets, and following dietary plans based on these concepts can result in an unbalanced diet and may actually interfere with peak athletic performance.

Besides being an unnecessary expense, megadoses of vitamin supplements taken inappropriately can also lead to nutritional imbalances and can endanger the athlete's health. A balanced diet is the best way to give the body pep and energy. Thus, athletes should follow a nutritious diet that emphasizes a variety of high-carbohydrate, lowfat foods.

Common Illnesses: Bacteria vs Viruses

Colds and other respiratory tract infections are common among athletes and can sideline an entire team if proper precautions are not taken. Contrary to what many believe, colds are primarily transmitted by touch, not by coughing and sneezing. These viruses are able to live for several days on hard surfaces, such as doorknobs, countertops, and equipment. All an athlete has to do to become infected is touch an infected surface and then transfer the virus to the respiratory system by rubbing the eyes or nose or touching the mouth.

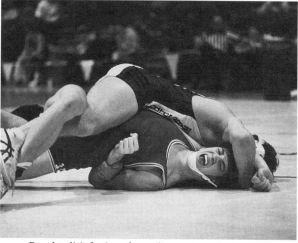

Regular disinfecting of wrestling mats and other equipment is the key to preventing the spread of skin diseases, such as herpes simplex.

As a student athletic trainer, you should remind athletes to be especially conscious about keeping their hands clean and keeping them away from the eyes and nose. Also, avoid the use of a community towel or drinking cup, as viruses can live on them as well.

Once an athlete has contracted a cold, there is no magic cure. Rest and light eating will generally be all that is necessary or helpful in treating the virus. Aspirin or non-aspirin pain relievers can minimize aching and discomfort by lowering fever. However, as a student athletic trainer, you are not the one who should dispense these medications.

The athlete must be fully recovered from a cold before returning to activity. Returning too soon can cause the virus to linger and possibly turn into a more serious illness.

Skin Conditions

There are a number of skin conditions that the athletic trainer will be exposed to during a typical sport season. These conditions will range from very minor to the medical emergency. The establishment of appropriate protocol for the handling of all skin conditions will make your job easier and the care given to your athletes more complete.

As with all conditions in which bodily fluids are present, you need to utilize latex gloves and follow the set of universal precautions in order to safeguard yourself in these matters. Additionally, the disposal of biohazardous waste must be done according to accepted guidelines of the local, state, and federal agencies.

Herpes Simplex

A common problem in sports, particularly among wrestlers, is the skin infection called herpes simplex. The virus, which can enter the body through breaks in the skin, can produce painful lesions anywhere on the body. Most often, a lesion will appear as a cold sore on the lip. Even after the disease subsides, the athlete will continue to be a carrier of the virus and will be susceptible to future attacks.

The danger of skin diseases such as herpes simplex is that they are highly contagious and can spread easily and rapidly to other members of the team. Another skin infection, impetigo, is similar in appearance to herpes simplex, but is much more contagious.

Treatment and isolation can help prevent the infection of other athletes. The student athletic trainer's jobs are to look for the first signs of skin lesions, to notify the physician and to keep equipment (especially wrestling mats) clean and disinfected.

Fungus Infections
Athlete's Foot (Tinea Pedis)

The spread of athlete's foot depends mainly on the individual athlete's susceptibility. But, as a team, your athletes can help prevent athlete's foot from spreading by following this program:
- Powder the feet daily.
- Dry the feet thoroughly after every shower, especially between and under the toes.
- Keep athletic shoes and street shoes dry by dusting them with powder daily.
- Wear clean sports socks and street socks daily.
- The shower and dressing rooms should be cleaned and disinfected daily.
- Athletes should use shower shoes (flip flops).

Once an athlete has become infected by the tinea pedis fungus, basic care includes the following:
- Keep the feet as dry as possible through the frequent use of foot powder.
- Wear clean, white socks to avoid reinfection, changing them daily.
- Use a standard fungicide for specific medication.

Jock Itch (Tinea Cruris)

Jock itch may be due to an actual fungal infection. Other conditions referred to as "jock itch" can result from an accumulation of moisture in the groin area or from the friction of athletic activity.

Jock itch appears as a brownish or reddish lesion in the groin area. The symptoms are mild to moderate itching, resulting in scratching and the possibility of a secondary bacterial infection. The

Common Medical Illnesses

In addition to skin conditions, the athletic trainer will be expected to evaluate for medical referral a number of medical illnesses. Once again, the range on these illnesses will be from mild to severe. The athletic trainer should realize his/her individual limitations and refer to the most appropriate health care provider when there is doubt as to the condition or treatment.

Heat Exhaustion - Not to be mistaken for heat stroke—Symptoms include dizziness, nausea, faintness, weakness - unconsciousness may follow. Skin pale, cool, moist, pulse rapid, respiration shallow and hurried.

Heat Stroke - Results from direct exposure to high temperatures especially in those taking alcoholic beverages or debilitated. Early symptoms are dizziness, weakness, nausea, spots before eyes and ringing in the ears. Skin: bright red, hot, dry. Rapid, strong pulse later becoming weak. Unconsciousness usually follows, temperature may reach 108 degrees.

Hypertension (High Blood Pressure)—Sustained elevated blood pressure, systolic 140, diastolic 90 in adults.

Hypothermia - Having a body temperature below normal. People with profound hypothermia may be assumed dead. Rewarming is the first order of treatment. Method depends on severity of hypothermia.

Abrasion - *A scraping away of a portion of skin or a mucous membrane as a result of injury or mechanical means.*

Incision - *A cut made with a knife.*

Laceration - *A wound or irregular tear of the flesh.*

Blister (Bullae) - *A bleb or vesicle containing fluid (serum, blood, pus), sometimes caused by pressure. (A collection of fluid below the epidermis).*

Burn - *Tissue injury resulting from excessive exposure to thermal, chemical, electrical, or radioactive agents. Classified as:*

    First Degree - *Superficial, damage being limited to outer layer of the epidermis. Characterized by erythema, hyperemia, tenderness, pain. No vesicles.*

    Second Degree - *Damage extends through the epidermis and into the dermis, but not of sufficient extent to interfere with regeneration of epidermis. Vesicles present.*

    Third Degree - *Both the epidermis and dermis are destroyed with damage extending into the underlying tissues. Tissue may be charred or coagulated.*

Puncture - *A hole or wound made by sharp pointed instrument.*

Sunburn - *Dermatitis due to exposure to the actinic (ultraviolet) rays of the sun.*

contagious spores of this fungus may be spread by direct contact, contaminated clothing or unsanitary locker rooms and showers. This fungus grows best in warm, moist, dark areas.

Jock itch should not be undertreated. If infection enters the area, the irritation can cause an athlete to miss days or even weeks of action. Powders, sprays and creams containing tolnaftate are best for treating jock itch. However, tolnaftate products are too powerful to be used as preventive means over an extended period of time. The best ways to prevent jock itch are to keep the area clean and dry and to use a lubricating ointment to lessen friction in the groin area. Avoid medications that are irritating or tend to mask the symptoms of a groin infection.

Infections that do not respond to normal treatment should be referred to the team physician.

Legal and Ethical Considerations

The world of athletics has recently experienced the same trend that other segments of society have dealt with—legal and ethical issues. The sports world is no longer immune to court cases and challenges by the legal system. Additionally, ethical standards are being examined and those involved with sport are being held to those standards.

Recreational Drugs

The increased use of "recreational drugs" (marijuana, cocaine, alcohol) by high school, college, and professional athletes has been recently exposed in the media, as well as the use of "performance-enhancing" agents (such as anabolic steroids and caffeine) by world-class performers.

This has led to another area of great concern, the abuse of chemical agents by the very young athlete. Besides possibly starting such an athlete down a road of chemical dependency, drug use can have serious and sometimes irreversible side effects.

Alcohol

This is the most commonly abused drug at all levels. The peer pressure to drink is extreme. Because of its universal acceptance in our society, alcohol remains the most difficult drug to control.

Alcohol, even taken after the contest, ultimately results in deterioration of the psychomotor skills of reaction time, eye-hand coordination, accuracy, balance, and complex coordination. Alcohol also impairs body temperature regulation, especially during prolonged exercise in cold environments. In addition, it consistently decreases strength, power, local muscular endurance, speed, and cardiovascular endurance.

Even though the athlete generally consumes alcohol in an attempt to gain psychological benefits, the psychomotor performance deteriorates first and most profoundly. Thus, the athlete ends up hurting, not helping, himself/herself.

Marijuana

Marijuana is the second most commonly abused substance by the young athlete. The athlete who uses marijuana, even on a casual basis, experiences very significant effects that have a direct bearing on athletic performance. These effects include:
Inhibition of the sweating mechanism in hot environments, which can lead to heat illness.

- Major impairment of coordination as measured by hand steadiness, body sway, and accuracy of execution of movement.
- Impairment of tracking performance, perceptual tasks, and vigilance.
- Slowed reaction time to visual and auditory stimuli.
- Altered perception of speed, time, and space.
- Short-term and long-term memory loss.
- Prolonged learning time.

Probably the most serious effect of marijuana on the very young athlete is the establishment of a characteristic set of personality changes seen in marijuana users. This "anti-motivational syndrome" is characterized by apathy, loss of ambition and effectiveness, diminished ability to carry out long-term plans, difficulty in concentrating, decline in academic and athletic performance, intermittent confusion, impaired memory and loss of energy.

Anabolic Steroids

Anabolic steroids, synthetic derivatives of the male hormone testosterone, are some of the most controversial drugs linked to athletics. What do athletes expect to gain by taking steroids? For the most part, they are hoping to increase their strength and the size of their muscles.

Commonly, athletes on steroids also feel more aggressive and self-confident, which encourages them to train harder. There have been additional claims that steroids will do everything from increase red blood cell counts to act as glycogen-sparing (or energy-sparing) agents. The problem is that there is little conclusive evidence concerning the benefits of steroid use. Researchers agree that when normal, healthy men take steroids without training, there is no effect on muscle size or strength.

The harmful side effects of steroid use have been much better documented than any strength gains. Among the side effects in males are liver damage (including liver cancer), impaired kidney function, enlargement of the prostate gland, decreased levels of natural testosterone, testicular atrophy resulting in sterility, growth of breast tissue, and weight gain caused by fluid retention which often leads to elevated blood pressure. Some of these side effects can even lead to death. In addition, the majority of athletes using steroids experience an increase in libido and in detrimental aggressive behavior. In women, steroids can produce a deepened voice, growth of facial and chest hair, liver damage, clitoral enlargement, menstrual irregularities, and impairment of reproductive capacity.

Caffeine

Moderate amounts of caffeine can increase mental alertness, but too much may cause anxiety and hamper performance. In endurance events lasting more than two hours, caffeine can enhance performance as it allows the body to burn more fatty acids as fuel. However, unless your athletes participate in marathons, caffeine probably will not give them an advantage.

In addition, beverages containing caffeine have a diuretic effect. They stimulate the flow of urine, which may cause discomfort during activity or decrease the body's water level before competition, adversely affecting performance.

Recognition of Drug Use

Spotting a drug user or abuser can be a difficult and complicated task for a coach, athletic trainer, or student athletic trainer. Some of the changes that may be seen in an athlete using drugs resemble the symptoms of severe personal or emotional problems. It is imperative to treat the athlete as an individual and to talk to him or her privately about the nature of the problem.

Signs of drug use include:
- Increase in motivation
- Change in personality or behavioral patterns
- Withdrawal from companionship
- Decline in performance, both physically and academically
- Frequent missing of classes, especially physical activity classes
- Inability to coordinate (standing or walking)
- Poor personal hygiene and grooming
- Muddled speech
- Impaired judgment
- Restless, jittery
- Muscular twitches, tremor of hands
- Heavy sweating, bad breath, nervousness (amphetamine abuse)
- Red eyes, listlessness, increased appetite with special craving for sweets (marijuana abuse)

Tobacco Products

Recently, national sport governing bodies have taken the position that tobacco products are detrimental to the athlete and to the sport. Therefore, rules and regulations have been enacted to curb the use of tobacco products by all persons associated with athletic participation.

Those tobacco products that have been identified as having a negative impact on the health of the athlete include all smoking (especially when inhaled), chewing, and snuff tobacco products. Case studies have shown that cancer is linked to the use of these products. The sport of baseball has seen the most recent regulations enacted to control the use of these products while at practice and/or in game situations.

Drug Education/Drug Testing

World class, professional, and college athletes have been drug tested for decades. This is an attempt to make the playing field as equal as possible for all participants.

The trend is now toward the high school athlete and those participating at the recreational levels. This has developed because performance enhancing drug use has become common at those levels. Another factor that has influenced this trend is the cost and reliability of drug tests.

As with all issues of drug testing, the key is to educate the participants as to the detrimental effects of drug use. Most claims as to the beneficial effects of drug use are exaggerated and myth. The best way to counter this is through proper education of the coaches, athletic trainers, athletes, and parents.

Chapter 13 - Review Questions

Completion:

1. Most fungus infections grow in an environment that is _____, _____ and _____.

2. The common cold virus is transmitted primarily by _____, not by _____ or sneezing.

3. Skin is made up of the _____ and the _____.

4. Massaging small amounts of _____ into a callused area helps to maintain _____.

5. The technical term for a soft corn is _____ _____.

6. Treatment of intertrigo includes cleaning the affected area and applying a medicated _____ that will prevent infection and act as a _____ agent.

7. Uninfected abrasions require (1) _____, (2) thorough cleaning with _____ and _____, and (3) application of a moist dressing.

8. The tetanus _____ enters the body as a spore, at which time it multiplies unless the athlete has been _____ by a tetanus toxoid.

9. _____ is not an accurate indicator of an athlete's need for fluid replacement.

10. The gradual process of becoming used to hot weather and cold weather workouts is known as _____. This process takes about _____ weeks.

11. _____ are much more important than salt in avoiding heat problems.

12. A fluid loss of as little as _____ percent of total body weight can adversely affect endurance and coordination.

13. Heat stroke is a medical _____.

14. Heat stroke is caused by the body's inability to _____ heat.

15. Shock is a result of the collapse of the body's _____ system.

16. Besides fluid replacement, two special concerns during cold weather workouts are _____ and _____.

17. Replacing _____ after heavy sweating is far more important than replacing _____.

18. _____ is probably the most important contributing factor in weight gain.

19. _____ is the number one abused drug in the United States.

Short Answer:

1. Why is high temperature and elevated humidity dangerous?

2. What factors cause heat stroke?

3. How can an athlete prevent becoming dizzy or weak during practice if they do not get a chance to snack beforehand?

4. What is a good example of a pre- and post-activity menu that is low in fat content?

5. How are colds primarily transmitted?

6. What can happen if an athlete returns to activity before fully recovering from a cold?

7. Why is Herpes Simplex a dangerous skin disease within a team?

8. What is an abrasion?

9. What are the symptoms of heat exhaustion?

10. What is the blood pressure of someone in shock?

11 At all levels, what is the most commonly abused drug?

12. What can too much caffeine intake do?

13. How would you care for athlete's foot?

14. What are the signs and symptoms of heat exhaustion?

15. What are the first aid procedures for heat stroke?

16. What are the progressive signs of hypothermia?

17. List 3 ways to help prevent a cold virus from spreading among team members.
    •
    •
    •

18. List 3 of the harmful side effects of steroid use.
    •
    •
    •

NOTES

GLOSSARY
I. Base or Root Words

Term	Meaning	Term	Meaning
aden	gland	mentra	womb
angeion	vessel	mnesis	memory
arteria	artery	musculus	muscle
arthron	joint	myelos	marrow
blepharon	eyelid	myo	muscle
bronchos	bronchus	myringa	eardrum
bursa	sac	nephros	kidney
cardia	heart	neuron	nerve
carpus	wrist	oophoros	ovary
cephale	head	ophthalmos	eye
chir	hand	opsis	sight
chole	bile	orchis	testicle
chondros	cartilage	orexis	appetite
coccyx	last spinal bone	osme	smell
colon	bowel	osteon	bone
colpos	vagina	otos	ear
core	pupil (of eye)	pathos	disease
corneus	cornea (of eye)	pectus	chest
costa	rib	pes	foot
coxa	hip	pharynx	throat (part)
cranium	skull	phasis	speech
cutis	skin	philia	love
cystis	bladder	phlebos	vein
dacryon	tear	phobos	fear
dactylos	finger	phonos	voice
derma	skin	phoreo	perspiration
diaphragma	diaphragm	plasso	formation
dipsa	thirst	plexis	stroke
emein	vomit	pneumon	lung
enteron	gut	podikos	foot
esophagus	gullet	proktos	anus or rectum
gala	milk	psyche	mind
ganglion	nerve knot	pyelos	kidney pelvis
gaster	stomach	pyloros	pylorus
genos	origin	ren	kidney
glossa	tongue	rhin	nose
gone	gonad	salpinx	Fallopian tube
hema	blood	sarx	flesh
hepar	liver	sperma	semen
hystera	womb	sphygmos	pulse
ileum	small intestine	splen	spleen
iris	Iris (of eye)	stoma	mouth
keras	cornea (of eye)	tenon	tendon
kinesis	movement	thorax	chest
lac	milk	thymos	thymos
larynx	throat	thyreos	thyroid
mamma	breast	traches	windpipe
mastos	breast	trichinos	hair
meninx	membrane	urina	urine
mens	mind	uterus	womb

II. Prefixes

Prefix	Meaning	Prefix	Meaning
a, an	without, lack of	kinesi	movement
ab	from, away from	leuco, leuko	white
ad	to	macro	large
ambi	both	mal	ill, bad
amphi	on both sides	megalo	great
ana	up, apart, across	melano	dark, black
ankylo	adhesion	meso	middle
ante, antero	before, in front	meta	change, transformation
anti	against		
apo	from	micro	small
auto	self	multi	many
bi	twice, double, two	myo, my	muscle
bio	life	neo	new
brachy	short	nephro	kidney
brady	slow	neuro	nerve
cata, kata	down	ob	in front of
circum	around	oligo	few
co, com, con	with	ortho	straight
contra	against, opposite	osteo	bone
cyano	blue	pachy	thick
cyto	cell	pan	all, every
dactyl	finger, toe	para	beside
de	away from	per	through
di	twice, double	peri	around
dia	through	platy	broad
dis	apart from, not	pluri	several
dys	difficult, bad	polio	gray matter
e, ex	out of, out from	poly	many
ecto	outer	post, poster	after, behind
em, en	in	pre	before, in front
endo	within	pro	before, in behalf of
epi	on, upon	proto	first
eso	inward	pesudo	false
eu	good, well	pyo	pus
exo	outside	quadri	four, four fold
extra	beyond, outside	re	back, again
hem, haem	blood	retro	backward
hemi	half	semi	half
hetero	unlike	sub	under, less than
homo	similarity	sum, syn	with, together
hydro	water	super	above, more than
hyper	over, above	supra	above, upon
hypo	less, under, below	tachy	fast
im, in	in, not	teno	tendon
infra	below	trans	through, across
inter	between	ultra	beyond, in excess
intra	within	uni	one
intro	into		
iso	equal		

III. Suffixes

Suffix	Meaning	Suffix	Meaning
able	ability	oma	tumor
ac, al	pertaining to	or	agent or person
algia	pain	osis	action or condition
cele	swelling	ostomy	cutting & leaving an opening
cle,cule, culum, culus		otomy	cutting into
		ous	material
ectasis	expansion	pathy	disease
ectomy	cutting out	phile	affinity for
emia	blood	phobia	fear or dread
er	agent or person	plasis	growth, formation
esis	action or condition	placty	moulding, forming
ia	action or condition	ptosis	lowered position
ible	ability	rrhagia	break forth
ic, ious	pertaining to	rrhaphy	a sewing
id	state or condition	rrhea	flowing, discharge
ist, ite	agent or person	rrhexis	rupture
itis	inflammation	scopy	inspection, look in
ity	quality	spasm	contraction
ium	diminutive	stasis	stopping
logy	study of	sthenia	strength or activity
m, ma	result of action	therapy	treatment
malacia	softening	tion	action or condition
mania	madness	tripsy	crushing
odynia	pain	trophy	nourishment
oid	resemblance	uria	referring to urine
olum, olus	diminutive	y	action or condition

IV. Terminology

A. ASSOCIATED PROFESSIONS

SPORTS MEDICINE--broad, very inclusive term that includes a wide variety of medical and paramedical personnel. A sample list includes physicians, exercise physiologists, athletic trainers, kinesiologists, physical therapists, health educators, physical educators, nutritionists, and many more.

ATHLETIC MEDICINE--that specific portion of sports medicine which deals with competitive athletics.

ATHLETIC TRAINING--the prevention, treatment, and rehabilitation of athletic injuries. Probably can best be defined by examining the role of the athletic trainer.

ACSM--American College of Sports Medicine

NATA--National Athletic Trainers Association

NSCA--National Strength and Conditioning Association

ANATOMY--the study of structure or form.

PHYSIOLOGY--the study of function.

OSTEOLOGY--study of the skeletal system.

KINESIOLOGY--the study of human movement.

B. ANATOMICAL DIRECTIONS & BODY PLANES

ANTERIOR or VENTRAL--the front of the body or body part.

POSTERIOR or DORSAL--the back of the body or body part.

MEDIAL--toward the midline of the body.

LATERAL--away from the midline of the body.

MID SAGITTAL or MEDIAN--divides the body into equal and symmetrical right and left halves.

**Lateral and Medial, Superior and Inferior are also used to indicate surfaces, as well as directions or positions.

DORSAL--upper surface (e.g. top of foot).

VENTRAL--bottom surface (opposite of dorsal).

PLANTAR--ventral aspect of the foot (sole of the foot).

PALMAR--ventral aspect of the hand (palm of the hand).

VOLAR--ventral aspect of the hand (more commonly used when describing the fingers).

SUPERIOR--toward the top of the body or body part.

INFERIOR--toward the bottom of the body or body part.

EXTERNAL or PERIPHERAL--means near the surface.

INTERNAL--refers to a deeper position.

EVERSION--turning the sole of the foot outward.

IV. Terminology - *continued*

B. ANATOMICAL DIRECTIONS & BODY PLANES - continued

INVERSION--turning the sole of the foot inward.

ELEVATION (up)--as in lifting the shoulder up.

DEPRESSION (down)--just the opposite as in lowering the shoulder.

PROTRACTION (forward)--as in bringing the shoulder forward.

RETRACTION (backward)--as in pulling the shoulder back and thus bringing the shoulder blades together.

PROXIMAL--nearest to the point of attachment, origin, or other point of reference.

DISTAL--farthest from a point of reference (opposite of proximal).

ORIGIN--the fixed end or attachment of muscle.

INSERTION--muscle attachment to a bone that moves.

MAJOR--Means greater or larger (Pectoralis Major)

MINOR-- Means lesser or smaller (Pectoralis Minor)

ACTION--in physiology, the motions or functions of a part or organ of the body.

HYPER--(prefix)--meaning too much. [e.g. HYPERventilation, HYPERextension]

ANATOMICAL POSITION--the neutral stance of the individual; standing, facing forward with arms at the sides and palms facing forward.

FLEXION--movement around a transverse axis in an anterior-posterior plane with the angle between the anterior aspects of the displaced parts becoming smaller, as in bending the forearm toward the arm at the elbow joint.

EXTENSION--is the reverse movement during which the angle between the anterior aspects of the displaced parts is increased as in moving the forearm away from the upper arm.

ABDUCTION--movement lateral away from the median plane around an anterior-posterior axis with the angle between the displaced parts becoming greater, as in lifting the arm sideward away from the body.

ADDUCTION--is the opposite movement, as in bringing the arm from a sideward position back toward the body and thus decreasing the angle.

ROTATION--is movement around a longitudinal axis which passes through a joint as in turning the palm of the hand up or down with the arm abducted.

CIRCUMDUCTION--is movement around the horizontal and longitudinal axis of a joint during which the distal end of the bone circumscribes the base of an imaginary cone and proximal end forms the apex, as in swinging the arms in a circle.

PRONATION--is medial rotation of the forearm, as in turning the palm of the hand downward.

SUPINATION--is lateral rotation of the forearm, as in turning the palm of the hand upward.

IV. Terminology - *continued*

C. ANATOMICAL STRUCTURES

ARTICULATION--a joint between bones. The manner of connecting by a joint.

CERVICAL--of the neck, especially the seven vertebrae in the neck.

LUMBAR--vertebral column extending from the twentieth through the twenty-fourth vertebrae. Low back.

THORACIC--portion of vertebral column extending from the eighth through the nineteenth vertebrae. Upper back.

SACRUM--a curved triangular element of the backbone.

COCCYX--the 4 rudimentary bones at lowest end of the backbone; the vestigial human tail.

BONE--a supportive rigid connective tissue consisting of an abundant calcified matrix enclosing many branched cells.

CARTILAGE--gristle, a white, semiopaque, non-vascular connective tissue composed of a matrix containing nucleated cells which lie in cavities or lacunas of the matrix.

DERMAL--pertaining to the dermis; cutaneous.

LIGAMENT--a band of flexible, tough, dense white fibrous connective tissue connecting the articular ends of the bones and sometimes enveloping them in a capsule.

MUSCLE--a tissue composed of contractile fibers or cells. A contractile organ composed of muscle tissue, affecting the movements of the organs and parts of the body.

JOINT CAPSULE, ARTICULAR CAPSULE, SYNOVIAL CAPSULE--a sac-xlike, fibrous membrane that surrounds a joint. Often including or interwoven with ligaments.

BURSA--a fluid-filled sac or saclike cavity that allows a muscle or tendon to slide over bone (thereby eliminating friction). [BURSAE--plural]

SESAMOID BONE--a small bone inplanted in a tendon (e.g. the patella).

NERVE--a bundle of nerve fibers, usually outside the brain or spinal cord.

TENDON--a band of dense fibrous tissue forming the termination of a muscle and attaching to a bone.

EPIPHYSIS--growth plate.

AXIAL SKELETON--composed of the bones of the skull, the thorax, and the vetebral column. These bones form the axis of the body.

APPENDICULAR SKELETON--consists of the bones of the shoulder and the upper extremities, and the hips and the lower extremities. These bones form the appendages and attach to the axial skeleton.

D. CLASSIFICATIONS OF INJURIES

ACUTE--quick onset, short duration.

CHRONIC--of long duration, repeating. In athletes, usually a neglected injury or one that has not responded to treatment.

CONGENITAL--existing before or at birth. Dating from, but not necessarily detected at birth.

SUBACUTE--relatively acute; a stage between acute and chronic; after the initial trauma.

IV. Terminology - *continued*

D. CLASSIFICATIONS OF INJURIES - continued

EXPOSED--a wound or injury involving a break in the skin.

UNEXPOSED--a wound or injury that does not break the skin.

INFECTION--the invasion of a host by organisms, such as bacteria, fungi, viruses, protozoa, or insects with or without manifest disease.

TRAUMA--wound or injury.

SYNDROME--group of typical symptoms or conditions that characterize a deficiency or disease.

INFLAMMATION--reaction of the body tissue to an irritant.

ABSCESS--a collection of pus in the body.

ANTISEPTIC--a substance which prevents the growth of bacteria.

EDEMA--swelling as a result of the collection of fluid in the connective tissue.

EFFUSION--escape of the fluid into a cavity (such as within a joint capsule).

ECCHYMOSIS--extravasation (escape into tissues) of blood; also the tissue discoloration caused by the extravasation of blood.

CREPITUS--grating sound produced by the contact of the fractured ends of bones.

ADHESION--a sticking together or binding of tissue fibers.

ABRASION--a spot denuded of skin, mucous membrane, or superficial epithelium by rubbing or scraping.

AVULSION--a forcible tearing or wrenching away of a part, as a polyp, a nerve, or a limb.

INCISION--in surgery, a cut made into the tissue or organ.

LACERATION--a tear, or a wound made by tearing. The act of tearing or lacerating.

PUNCTURE--a hole made in the skin by the piercing of a pointed instrument.

BURSITIS--inflammation of a bursa.

DERMATITIS--inflammation of the skin.

CHRONDROMALACIA--softening of a cartilage.

CONCUSSION--shock; the state of being shaken; a severe shaking or jarring of a part, as by an explosion, or a violent blow.

CONTUSION--a bruise; an injury usually caused by a blow in which the skin is not broken.

CYST--an enclosed space within a tissue or organ, lined by epithelium and usually filled with fluid or other material.

LESION--Any local abnormality; bruise, wound, tumor or cavity, etc.

BENIGN-- Harmless

MALIGNANT--Dangerous; tending to produce death.

IV. Terminology - *continued*

D. CLASSIFICATIONS OF INJURIES - continued

DISLOCATION--the displacement of one or more bones of a joint, or of any organ from the original position.

SEPARATION--injury to a generally non-movable joint.

EPISTAXIS--nosebleed.

EXOSTOSIS--a benign cartilage; capped protuberance from the surface of long bones, but also seen on flat bones; due to chronic irritation as from infection, trauma, or osteoarthritis.

FRACTURE--the breaking of a bone or cartilage.

HEAT CRAMPS--a heat exposure syndrome characterized by hard work in heat, sweating heavily, and inadequate electrolytes intake. Usually manifested by spasms in arms, legs, and abdomen. Treatment normally includes ice, fluids, and foods containing sodium chloride.

HEAT EXHAUSTION--a heat exposure syndrome characterized by weakness, vertigo, headache, nausea, and peripheral vascular collapse, usually precipitated by physical exertion in a hot environment.

HEAT STROKE--a heat exposure syndrome characterized by a high fever (hyperpyrexia) and loss of sweating.

HEMATOMA--a circumscribed extravascular collection of blood, usually clotted, which forms a mass.

HERNIA--the abnormal protusion of an organ, or a part, through the containing wall of its cavity, usually the abdominal cavity, beyond its normal confines.

HEMATURIA--passing of blood in the urine.

HEMORRHAGE--escaping of blood through ruptured walls of vessels.

-ITIS--an inflammatory disease of (suffix).

MYOSITIS--inflammation of muscle tissue

MYOSITIS OSSIFICANS--inflammation of muscle, with formation of bone.

NECROSIS--Death of tissue or cells

OSGOOD SCHLATTERS--osteochondrosis of the tuberosity of the tibia, seen especially in adolescents. (Inflammation of both bone and cartilage.)

OSTEOCHONDRITIS DISSECANS--a joint characterized by partial or complete detachment of a fragment or articular cartilage and underlying bone.

PARALYSIS--loss of power of voluntary motion.

SCAR TISSUE--the hard fibrous type of tissue formed as a result of the healing of a wound or tear or pull.

SPUR--an outgrowth of bony tissue into muscles or skin.

SPRAIN--a wrenching of a joint, producing a stretching or laceration of the ligaments.

STRAIN--excessive stretching or overuse of a part, as of tendon/muscle.

TENOSYNOVITIS--inflammation of a tendon and its sheath.

ASPIRATION--the withdrawing of fluids and gases from a cavity.

IV. Terminology - *continued*

E. THERAPEUTIC EXERCISE

CAST--to produce a specific form by pouring material (metal, plaster, etc.) into a prepared mold.

SURGERY--the branch of medicine dealing with trauma and diseases requiring operative procedure.

SUTURE--a fine thread or cord-like material used to make a repair or close a wound.

AEROBIC--work requiring oxygen.

ANAEROBIC--work not requiring oxygen.

EXERCISE--muscular exertion for the purpose of preservation or restoration of health or development of physical prowess or athletic skill.

ATROPHY--decrease in muscle or tissue size.

HYPERTROPHY--enlargement of a part caused by an increase in the size of its cells.

ISOMETRIC--static. Contraction of a muscle without movement. A muscular contraction in which the muscle fibers do not shorten in length resulting in no movement of adjoining body parts. Muscle works with no change in muscle length. Builds static strength, but does not improve dynamic strength significantly.

ISOTONIC--dynamic; e.g. weight lifting. A muscular contraction in which the muscle fibers shorten in length resulting in movement of the adjoining body parts. Muscle works with a change in muscle length.
   Concentric--shortening
   Eccentric--lengthening

ISOKINETIC--dynamic. A form of isotonic exercise in which the possibility of maximum resistance can be provided through the full range of movement. Muscle works with a change in muscle length and controlled speed. Requires an accomodating resistance device, e.g. a Mini-Gym.

CONCENTRIC--refers to muscle shortening.

ECCENTRIC--refers to muscle lengthening.

F. THERAPEUTIC MODALITY

MODALITY--method or apparatus for therapy.

PALPATION--examination by touch.

INDICATE--to advise a particular treatment.

CONTRAINDICATE--to warn against a particular treatment.

LOCAL--particular to a certain area.

CRYOTHERAPY--treatment by use of cold.

CRYOKINETICS--treatment combining cold and exercise.

THERAPY--treatment of diseases or injuries.

HYDROTHERAPY--treatment by use of water (whirlpools for example).

IV. Terminology - *continued*

F. THERAPEUTIC MODALITY - continued

WHIRLPOOL--a bath in which an arm or a leg or greater part of the body is immersed in water (hot or cold) which is agitated by a whirling or churning current of equally water (hot or cold) mixed with air.

HYDROCOLLATOR--moist heat packs.

MASSAGE--the act of rubbing, kneading, or stroking the superficial parts of the body with the hand or with an instrument.

ANALGESIC--a counterirritant which reduces pain and increases local circulation.

THERMOTHERAPY--treatment by use of heat (hot packs, analgesics, ultrasound, and diathermy are all included).

DIATHERMY--the use of electrical current to increase circulation by heating.

ULTRASOUND--the use of sound waves to produce heating in the tissues.

ELECTRICAL STIMULATION--the use of an electrical current, either alone or with another modality to reduce muscle spasm.

INFRARED--invisible heat rays beyond the red end of the electromagnetic spectrum, used as a superficial heat modality.

ULTRAVIOLET--invisible light rays, most commonly associated with sun burns, used as a superficial heat modality.

TRACTION--the act of drawing or pulling.